How to use th

CW01020247

Obviously this book can be
but its true intention is to p
weekly inspiration for prac
inspiration, a theme can be ..... .,..
day's practice. It is by bringing the study of Tai
Chi into practice, that advancement is possible.
Proceeding in this fashion systematically week
by week, the various areas of study related to
the Tai Chi form can be addressed and clarified.
As the old saying goes, "If only the 形 Xing
(form) is practiced and not the 功 Kung (skill), in
the end all that will be produced is embroidered
feet and flowery hands. This is a warning. Don't
simply go through the movements in a mindless
rote fashion, but with a clear objective of the
day's work ahead; what flaws need attention,
and an enthusiastic applied work ethic to
amplifying an existing skill level. Tai Chi is not
an atheistic dance that adorns the body like
fancy embroidered shoes and flashy jazz hands.
Students must beware the perils of the path,
where a dull boring practice breeds lethargy, or
lack of mental clarity spawn frustration from a
confused mind.
It is possible to learn rudimentary Tai Chi from a
book or video, if no teacher is available, but this
is not that book. This book is meant to be used in
association with a realized instructor. This book
may create more questions than offer concrete
resolutions, but this is advantageous to a deeper
study. Tai Chi is a "mind directed" engagement.
Ultimately, we teach ourselves with the guidance
of a superior. A good teacher is a person who
can explain a complex subject in simple
understandable terms. A good student is not a
baby, opening its mouth waiting to be feed, but
grabs for the spoon eager to feed themselves.
There is no limit to learning. It is up to the

student to decide how deep they desire to go down the rabbit hole and emerge victorious. After reading a weekly lesson, students are encouraged to seek other resources and research the material in greater depth. After being presented a year's worth of direction, students should pick up the mantle themselves and craft their own destiny. Tai Chi is vast. Destinations are not set in stone. Constantly evaluating the path under the feet, can make the journey more fruitful. A teacher is merely a finger pointing at the moon. Don't miss your own voyage, by staring too closely at the teacher's finger. Additionally, a hair off target, we will completely miss the moon. Be clear yourself. Considering Tai Chi can be pursued as a method of Self-Defense, a means for maintaining health as a therapeutic exercise, or a cultivation practice toward spiritual attainment, a multidimensional view of the hand form can create a journey to last a lifetime. Traditionally, as students of the Tao (Way) of Tai Chi, we progress from warrior to healer to sage. A warrior protects all life. A healer seeks to cure the dis-ease of suffering in themselves and by extension, offers aid to those in need. A sage shares a lifetime of wisdom for the benefaction of the world.

It is this author's hope that readers will find the information and resources presented here to empower their own study and practice. To seek refuge in a higher power of their own choosing, the world in which they live, and the vast ocean of knowledge available. Not by relying on others to do the work for them, but by their own efforts; continuously giving back more, than they received. In this way, we will all continue to advance. Leaving behind something greater to our progeny, than was received by our ancestry.

Week 1 - Exercise

Youth engage in exercise mainly as a means to improve body aesthetics and performance in sport competitions. Health is usually not their major objective. Generating greater aerobic endurance, often done by running fast, where the sustained motion of the body causes the heart to pump faster (cardiovascular system), supplying oxygenated blood via the breathing action of the lung (respiratory system) or through resistance training like weight lifting, that places a greater demand on the muscular system to handle increasingly heavier weight, bolsters strength and crafts a shapelier body with toned muscles.

As we age, it is not that this form of exercise needs to be completely abandoned, but health issues and sustained wear and tear on aging body parts becomes a consideration in engaging in such dynamic pursuits. Therapeutic exercise seeks to be safe to avoid injury (Do no harm) by clearly addressing existing health problems, body usage limitations, and provide motivation to sustain practice to proactively work toward graceful aging that keeps the quality of life abundant year after year.

To accomplish this, it is important that exercise be enjoyable and sustainable. Pushing hard, creating muscular strain, and mental frustration to gain a conceptualized benefit quicker, is to swim against the current. The body and mind become adversaries to overcome. Working at an appropriate, personally modified level creates a relaxed mental / physical state, like floating down stream and acquiring the benefits along the way at a leisurely pace. The body and mind become allies in addressing the inevitable weaknesses that manifest over time, instead of enduring a life of inactivity, hardship, and unresolvable pain.

As a therapeutic exercise the Tai Chi hand form should be approached as a practice of relaxed, balanced, continuous motion, instead of a collection of fixed specific postures that the body must be forced to assume perfectly. By making the body shape (known as the frame) softer and less expansive, a "Place of Power" can be established. Erroneously moving into one uncomfortable, tight, and unsustainable posture after another will not nurture our health. Conceptualizing and trying to do it right, is definitely not the same as experiencing and feeling if it is right for "your" body. The creation of tension and instability is very tangible for everybody. The form's standardized choreography provides a transitory venue to study how the body works in articulation. Just like a child learns to stand and walk, we as adults take a "Backward Step" to observe and correct what we usually take for granted. By "Investing in loss"; taking the time to improve the quality of what we already have and addressing our weaknesses directly, we conserve rather than waste our energies and feel the results intimately.

Week 2 - Path

At various times in our lives, we resolve to embrace change to solve a problem or more proactively prevent a situation from ever manifesting. Regardless of our actions, it is important to realize time never stops and change is relentless. Like rust, it never sleeps. The best we can hope to do is maintain or improve our lives by slowing the moment to moment effects of atrophy.

With careful thought, we choose a path that hopefully will lead us in our intended direction. Once the decision is made, it is our consistent perseverance and applied effort that will send us down the road. Although tangents may lead us astray periodically along our journey, returning to the path will continue to guide us to unlimited destinations and reap undreamed of rewards.

The path must be actualized daily, for no amount of good intentions can produce the benefit. Don't put off for tomorrow, what can be done today should be resolute. It is said, **"One day of practice provides that day with a benefit."** It cannot be banked to spend on days off the path. Although what actually takes place, is each day's engagement produces a more effective and efficient practice. Twenty minutes...for the beginner is spent finding their energy...for the intermediate is spent developing their energy...for the advanced student is spent refining their energy. Like obtaining a medicinal purified elixir, a little can do a lot daily.

To make this Path analogy crystal clear, we are traveling through time, not necessarily space. Every day at a specific hour I may practice in my regular place, but I am not the same. Although I may move within a small area of 10 feet square, I have journeyed countless miles in practice. Each time is a new and fresh adventure. The point is, we cannot simply absent mindedly wander down a garden path. We must be fully aware of everything and grasp at its full potential daily.

We usually fail to realize our objectives because we do not stick to the path. We must study to gain the theories and principles of Tai Chi that once applied to our bodies through practice will generate the energies that transforms us daily. We change due to the very journey we create by our own efforts of study and practice.

Although we may support each other, the journey must be made alone. The teacher's finger points to the moon. Each student must make the trip themselves. The true path is difficult and lonely only to those who do not know themselves. Only you can go into the darkness found inside your body and illuminate it. A teacher can only make corrections to the external flaws they observe and detect, the student must relate these pointers to the internal world they experience through "Sensation" and breathe fresh life into their practice. Don't "Just do it". Feel it. Be it. Live it.

The two pillars of learning are Study and Practice. Study is academic and dogmatic. We seek to comprehend the knowledge of those accomplished masters who preceded us in the past. Before we can discriminate and draw educated conclusions, we need to gather sufficient information about the subject. It is very difficult to play both roles of teacher and student. Unfortunately, as students we tend not to listen to direction, disregarding steps we feel unnecessary or laborious, while gravitating toward studies we find easy and feel confident. It is said, "Best to learn it right the first time" as to be more efficient with time / resources and progress expediently. Often it may be better to do the things we need to do, rather than want to do.

Study involves memorization. Classically this was done verbally by rote. The teacher spoke and all the students replied, or an individual was asked to recite information from a posed question. Memorization of information is critical to practice. The student may only attend an hourly class once or thrice a week to learn, but it is the time spent in solitary practice that is of the highest importance. The master saxophonist Charlie Parker stated, "It is not only how long and hard you practice, but what you practice". Study is simply to know what to practice.

Regardless if a student performs correctly or not, if after the execution they can recognize their mistakes and understand why they occurred, then through a mindful practice the flaw can be reduced and eventually eliminated. Without such knowledge of correctness, the student is doomed to solidify their mistakes, which at a later time are extremely difficult to uproot and remove. We say, "Practice the Gong (Skills), not the Form". Due to the fact Form follows Function, if one mindlessly moves through the form and does not apply their acquired knowledge to improve the skills used to create the form, in the end the student will only have embroidered feet and fancy hands. This means the form will be merely an aesthetic dance lacking the energy development of the body that produces the therapeutic effect. In solo practice, if you don't know what to do...do what you know.

Reading books, watching videos, attending class and seminars, asking questions, and investigating collateral subjects like anatomy, physics, psychology, etc. are all avenues to increase knowledge about Tai Chi. This is the scholarly aspect applying Mind over Matter that provides the food to fuel the physical practice. Directing the body with the mind, is the primary action of every physical movement. Expressed as "Mind first, Body second." or practically as "Look before you leap."

Tai Chi is simply a study of how the body functions in movement. In the next installment, we will address how to put this knowledge into physical practice.

The two pillars of learning are Study and Practice. Practice is a somatic, practical, hands - on and pragmatic experience. It is important to consider the mind of knowledge is stored in the brain which is a "physical" organ of perception. The mind is the body. The body is the mind. The mind directs the body's functions via the central nervous system. The nervous system that operates automatically is called the Autonomic nervous system, but the system we use to practice via mindful control over the body is called the Somatic nervous system.

We often take for granted the almost magical ability we possess to move our bodies at will, until due to advancement of age, injury or disease our bodies cannot respond at all, or to our satisfaction at sufficient dexterous levels. Tai Chi as a form of conscious movement practice aims to restore and improve the body's usage not by only focusing on the physical articulation of the torso and limbs, but also the whole human organism used to initiate and sustain movement. This includes addressing both uncomfortable and pleasant physical sensations along with the associated fluctuating emotional states that arise during practice in the mind too.

In motion, for every action, there will be a reaction. Physical practice is to be mentally aware of the sensations generated in the body. The skill of shifting moves the centerline of the body and changes the weight distribution. This can be considered an action that will result in standing on one leg. The reaction is, was the action successful? Did the action create stability? What sensations were generated in motion?

It is important to develop a temperament of equanimity. To simply deal with physical sensations for what they are and not elevate them into negative emotions. Without training, a slight imbalance can cause an overreaction, where anxiety (to achieve balance) and fear (from loss of balance) increase to the point of loss of control. In challenging yourself, maintaining calm will help the body stay relaxed and manageable. When balancing on one leg, if central equilibrium is lost, it is better to gently fall and touch the foot to the ground regaining control, rather than breaking with Tai Chi principles; tightening muscles to brace in an attempt to hold a posture.

Considering the high level of internal attention, cloistered solitary practice becomes a form of moving meditation. Once brought to proficiency, public performance offers an opportunity to practice a higher level of mind - body integration. Initially, the student uses the memorization of the standardized form as one-point concentration. Later various themes focusing on specific aspects of applied theory to different body parts become the objective of each practice session. The mind's knowledge directs the body's action. The body's reaction is felt as sensation.

We experience the body through a conscious appreciate of the sensations it produces via the five sense organs. The eyes are sensitive to light, the nose sensitive to odor, the tongue sensitive to flavor, the ears sensitive to tones, and the body's sensitivity to external and internal stimulation referred to as touch or feeling. Tai Chi as a whole body practice seeks to gain greater sustained conscious awareness of the body's ever changing sensations. If a sensation is conceptualized and deemed pleasant or uncomfortable, thinking about it further and discriminating in terms of like or dislike, good or bad creates a separate cerebral idea about the sensation that is very different than an intimate "Mind in the Body" physical feeling.

When we attempt to learn something new and challenge our existing level of ability, which is a continuous case as we pursue higher and higher levels of physical dexterity, the body devoid of conscious sensation (known as body awareness) often responds automatically beyond our control by tightening, especially when we are not clear on how to precede exactly and try to forcefully accomplish the objective at any cost. The mind's focused direction is the key to working with the body's sensations. It should be noted; the mind is sensitive to the very thoughts the brain produces from the information received from the other five sense organs. Overloaded with distracting and tangent agendas, when entertaining every random irrelevant thought, it is impossible to be fully present in the body. What we are seeking is a unified experience of the mind in the body and body in the mind. When we stop to reflect mentally as the body continues on its course, it is like a ship without a Captain at the helm. The conscious body unites. Mind Body One. The reflective mind separates. Mind in mind. Discursive thought blinds the eye of perception.

Moving the body slow and steady allows us ample time to feel even the minutest fluctuation in our body. Possibly responding quickly enough to a small imperfection and "nipping it in the bud" before it grows out of control. It is certainly more challenging to do Tai Chi slow because it requires a higher degree of moment to moment mental concentration and a willingness to experience the flaws instead of rush past them. We must experience many uncomfortable states like loss of balance and stiffness, prior to feeling more favorable comfortable states like rock solid stability and ease of motion, if we strive to improve rather than just do. The point to realize is, that if we strive continuously toward correctness, and incrementally amplify our skills through measured challenges, we will reach higher plateaus. By listening to what the body is trying to tell us through sensation and yielding to its wisdom, rather than pushing through with the mind's forceful intentions, we are working with the body. We are in the body. Absolute and at one with ourselves.

Outside the body using the light of day, we can see the body's shape and discern its strengths and weakness, but inside the body it is dark like night. We must use the mind's eye and inner vision to penetrate into this mysterious internal landscape. The mind must be in the body and the body must be in the mind.

Mind in Body - The study and practice of Tai Chi is both conceptual and visceral. It is an endless cycle of filling the mind with recallable technical knowledge and actualizing it out daily in the body as tangible motion studies. A clear mental picture of the body is truly worth a thousand words to the mind. If it is possible to visualize it, recreating it is feasible. Imagination becomes reality. For example, a front bow stance requires: heels shoulders width apart, front foot straight, back foot 45 degrees, front knee bent over metatarsals, rear knee straight but not locked, 70% front and 30% rear leg weight distribution, while maintaining central equilibrium. If this is not clear in the mind, how is it possible to evaluate sufficient from deficient cause and effect? In this respect, time in class with the teacher is for learning by asking questions and observing demonstrations. The most rewarding practice is done alone. It is a time to try to actualize the lesson and reinforce previous acquired skills gained through an applied study. Regular practice often leads to comprehension and seeking advanced knowledge. Irregular practice leads to frustration and stagnation due to the difficulty of mentally recalling the lessons.

Body in Mind - Once the body is placed into a posture following the mind's instructions, a teacher can evaluate its outer shape for irregularities and correctness. Although it is the student alone that feels the posture. Often in learning a new movement we feel awkward or unnatural. This is simply because the inner shape does not match the often forced outer shape. Here the teacher must explain what they feel inside their own dark body. How they manipulate their structure to create a relaxed and balanced form, rather than strain and brace to hold an idealized posture. Physical sensation is the key. By making the shape smaller and not locking joints, tension is reduced. By using alignment, relaxation, and upward energy a flexible sustainable balanced posture results because the student made the shape appropriate for their own body. The point is not to just try to copy and reproduce a perceived correct shape, but to feel that a shape is correct because it seeks to maintain relaxation and balance in the body and is conducive to movement. The mind is always moving, the shape is always changing, yin and yang are constantly exchanging. There is no permanence except for the moment to moment pursuit to maintain functional relaxation and balance in the continuous motion of the hand form's performance. See the whole body. Feel the whole mind.

There are three topics that should be studied and brought into practice to improve balance. Alignment, Relaxation, and Upward Energy. Regardless if balancing in a static position or balance related to movement, balance is an active process and should not be thought of as bracing or holding a fixed posture with muscular tension. Maintaining balance continuously and consistently is reliant on the mind's awareness to respond appropriately to small physical changes inside the body (inner awareness) and also in the surrounding environment (outer attention).

Part 1- Alignment

The location of the feet on the ground forms the body's Base of Support. When the body is positioned within this base of support, bearing the body's entire weight correctly there is stability. When the body is moved outside this base, by erroneous actions like leaning and over reaching, loss of balance occurs.

Length - Starting in the Prepare Stance with the feet parallel, weight is distributed in the foot between the ball pad and heel pad by moving the Centerline (Perineum to Crown) forward and backward. Placing slightly more weight (60%) in the ball pad and the remaining weight (40%) in the heel pad is conducive to better balance. Standing directly over the ankles causes dysfunctional compression of the ankle joint. In a Bow Stance, by moving the Centerline forward and backward weight can be shifted to the front or rear leg.

Width - The weight of the body can be supported totally on either leg, or in varying proportions between the two legs. In the Prepare Stance, shifting the Centerline laterally (left and right) between the two legs determines which leg bears the bulk of the weight. Placed directly in the center, each leg supports 50% of the body's weight. Moving the Centerline closer to one leg, it is possible to place 100% of the weight on that leg (Yang / Substantial / Full), while the other leg bear no weight at all (Yin / Insubstantial / Empty).

Height - Working with gravity, the feet, legs, spine, neck, and head form the body's vertical axis (up and down). The shoulders and pelvis (hips) are the body's horizontal axis (left and right). The posterior and anterior (front and back). Leaning in any horizontal direction causes loss of Central Equilibrium and Upward Energy pitching the weight in that direction causing a feeling of instability from imbalance.

Being mentally aware (conscious) of physical sensation is key to alignment. To understanding this academically and experience it pragmatically is to study and practice Balance.

There are three topics that should be studied and brought into practice to improve balance. Alignment, Relaxation, and Upward Energy. Regardless if balancing in a static position or balance related to movement, balance is an active process and should not be thought of as bracing or holding a fixed posture with muscular tension. Maintaining balance continuously and consistently is reliant on the mind's awareness to respond appropriately to small physical changes inside the body (inner awareness) and also in the surrounding environment (outer attention).

Part 2 - **Relaxation**

The Chinese term used for relaxation is Song. Although it is not the limp, lethargic attitude associated with motionless rest, but an active form that attempts to maintain a moving posture that is neither too tight, restricting freedom of motion, or too limp, collapsing the body's structure necessary for stability. The lower body (legs) and upper body (torso and arms) need to be addressed separately because their function is different, but they must be harmonized together to be fully functional.

The legs support the body's weight. Misaligned, muscles must brace forcefully to stabilize the structure. Like an improperly built house, instead of "dropping the weight" of the roof into the foundation through the framework, poor design and craftsmanship creates compromised spots that "hold up" too much weight. The downward forces get trapped and eventually the framework gives way under the excessive strain. Instead of thinking of building fixed solid stances, it is more appropriate in continuous motion, to think of moving into and out of constantly changing pliant supportive frames that meet the requirements to maintain balance and relaxation. If the body is forced to assume a conceived idealized shape with the loss of these requirements, undue tension and restrictive movement results.

The upper body sits on the legs. The lower body is heavy like a jade table. Even in motion it feels rooted to the ground. The legs are always under the compression of the torso's weight. When this weight is properly managed from below, the upper body can "relax down". Upper muscles relax making the body feel light and free to move. Often when the lower body fails to do its job correctly, to compensate and maintain stability upper muscles are tightly braced. This is referred to as "Raising up the Chi" (energy) and activating muscles that do not need to be energized.

When the body tightens erroneously causing loss of Song (relax) this loss of ease of motion (internal restriction) requires more force to move the body. This increased force often leads to loss of balance. The body is being forcefully pushed off its foundation instead of being allowed to relax down (sink) and move effortlessly.

There are three topics that should be studied and brought into practice to improve balance. Alignment, Relaxation, and Upward Energy. Regardless if balancing in a static position or balance related to movement, balance is an active process and should not be thought of as bracing or holding a fixed posture with muscular tension. Maintaining balance continuously and consistently is reliant on the mind's awareness to respond appropriately to small physical changes inside the body (inner awareness) and also in the surrounding environment (outer attention).

Part 3 – **Upward Energy**

Typical to any Yinyang discussion we must speak in terms of complimentary opposites. To understand upward energy known as Fun Kai (open and expand), we must address downward energy known as Song (relax and sink) too. Just like a car jack must be on an unyielding foundation to lift a car up, the body must be rooted to the Earth to expand freely up to the Heavens.

If the body is too limp, the fascia and joints are compressed restricting free articulation. Generating a greater force is required to sustain movement by pushing through these restrictions which often results in imbalance. If the body is properly supported from below by the legs and feet, the upper body can open upward making it light and agile. The 24 vertebra of the spine are supple and easily aligned responding to the body's gravity attraction with Earth, which is a major consideration in consistent balance. It should be clearly noted here that the spine is never in a fixed position that must always remain vertically straight, but when folded and closed properly (like forming a letter C shape) as in squatting, it continuously adjusts to maintain an alignment (Central Equilibrium) that is conducive to sustained balance. Continuous balance in motion is created by the upper body's mass always being properly supported by the base of support (legs and feet).

"Raising a light, lively, and intangible energy to the top of the head" is a mentally induced upward expansion of the body that is fully aware of maintaining a body that is not too limp or not too tight and rooted to the Earth. Muscular tightness is caused when instead of allowing the fascia to open freely by using proper joint aliment and inducing a relaxed feeling throughout the movement with the mind, absent mindedly crude muscular force is employed. It is this tension that braces the body in a tight fixed position that is destructive to balance. Instead of being relaxed and sunk into the Earth, the body seems to float on its root and topples over easily. The body lost its pliancy and ability to respond effortlessly. In an extreme locked open or closed state, the body must unlock first to reestablish its true foundation.

3-Dimensional Exercise

To change the weight distribution on the feet (Base of Support), move the Centerline (perineum to crown) while maintaining a vertical alignment (Central Equilibrium) by shifting the waist (horizontal alignment) using the legs and feet.

Prepare Stance - Feet parallel, heels shoulders distance apart, weight distribution is 50% on each leg, with 60% ball pads and 40% heel pads across both feet.

Horizontal Plane

1) **Length** - Shift the waist forward and backward moving the Centerline.

Practice:

Shift the waist backward. 50% weight on each heel pad and drum the ball pads.

Shift the waist forward. 50% weight on each ball pad and lift the heel pads.

Massage the feet by Shifting the waist back and forth from heel pads to ball pads.

2) **Width** - Lateral left to right Centerline movement.

Practice: Shift the waist so the weight is 100% on one foot then the other.

Vertical Plane

3) **Height** - upward energy from feet to perineum to crown of head.

Keep the body's Centerline upright and perpendicular to the Base of Support.

Remember if the Centerline moves while standing on one foot, you will lose balance and need unnecessary force/tension to stabilize.

Practice: Standing on one foot for longer periods of time

Inward and outward foot circles (ankle)

Knee (hip) and foot (ankle) lifts

Open the Door (Open the "Kua" - crotch laterally)

Upper leg (hip), lower leg (knee), and foot (ankle) stepping extensions

Knee circles (hip)

In Tai Chi theory, there are two main principles of Yinyang interaction, emergent and symbiotic. Viewing everything in a constant state of change or coming into being is called emergence. This is categorized as alternating cycles of creation (Yang) and destruction (Yin). Although these pairs may be subjectively viewed as good or bad, objectively they are a natural occurrence like life (Yang) and death (Yin). Seeing things for what they truly are and not just what we desire is key.

Most of us today live full hectic lives. Often scheduling plans far in advance yearly, monthly, or weekly. Our day is usually a timeline of hourly appointments, deadlines, or tasks that need to be done expeditiously. No wonder we are always stressed out from the anxiety to complete our endless daily agendas, or from the internal pressure we live under created by the fear from the repercussions if we fail.

The Tai Chi Form practiced as a method of moving meditation can train the student to use their mind and body in an enlightened way that can be brought into their everyday lives. People who are active in alcohol and substance abuse recovery programs are encouraged to "take it one day at a time". Although this is a good way to reduce anxiety about the future, in meditation we take it further to "second by second". When the mind is trained to fully absorb in the present task at hand, there is no separation of body and mind, where the student is off daydreaming about past and future events while the body is engaged in activity.

Being in the body and not lost in discursive thought, but experiencing the immediate sensations that arise and fall, paying attention to what is really happening from our actions, and responding appropriately, instead of forcing a favored outcome is the path to deeper relaxation. By removing the anxiety of failure, a student can correct what is restricting their progress, rather than trying to succeed at any cost.

We are always dealing with our body's gravitational attraction to the Earth through balance. When we align ourselves with it, there is no need to tighten and brace the body for stabilization. A muscularly relaxed body functions more efficiently under less stress. By directly dealing with the reality of a situation in the present moment we are in control. This empowers the mind and body. If while standing on one leg we sense imbalance, we try to realign. If you begin to fall, we don't panic furthering the tension that hastens our downward collapse, but relaxing we place the foot on the floor reestablishing our composure. It is best to minimize the damages and realize things will go wrong. Stressing out is not the answer. Staying present and relaxed in the midst of constant change leads to effective and efficient resolution.

To accept the emergent world is to see our symbiotic relationship with it. As things ceaselessly change, we respond accordingly and "go with the flow". This does not imply we a rudderless boat, adrift as a victim on the merciless sea, but on the contrary, as Sun Tzu points out in his book, The Art of War we have the potential to ride the waves and navigate through rough seas.

"If you know the enemy and know yourself, you need not fear the result of a hundred battles. If you know yourself but not the enemy, for every victory gained you will also suffer a defeat. If you know neither the enemy nor yourself, you will succumb in every battle."

Stress is often a result from the fear of the unknown. When faced with a barrier, our options are only fight or flight. When we choose to become the barrier and see it as ourselves this separation is dissolved. Studying and practicing Tai Chi is to realize the symbiotic nature of our internal body in movement and our external reactions in relationship to our external environment. By shoring up our perceived weaknesses, we empower ourselves.

Being centered mentally and physical promotes feeling balanced and in control. Central Equilibrium (height: **center** - up and down) is a symbiotic relationship that constantly maintains its position in association with length (**front** and **back**) and width (**left** and **right**). Note, fundamentally these **5 Directions** are always present in standing and motion because we exist in three dimensions. When we lose this symbiotic relationship (not living dimensionally), for example by creating an over expansive forward motion (weight in the front toes) while destroying our root in the back foot (heel leaving the floor), a loss of balance occurs. The physical occurrence of excessive tension (bracing to stop falling forward) is a result of an internal automatic reaction of the autonomic nervous system that strives to protect the body. A common military statement, "Stay alert, stay alive" hammers this home.

Stress produced by everyday use of the body can be greatly reduced by strengthening the Somatic nervous system through the motion studies provided by practicing the Tai Chi form. In this safe practice medium, the student can explore and experiment with the extremes of their capacities and reduce the overreaction caused when loss of control occurs. Instead of panic due to a sudden ballistic change, by being in control of movement and being mentally aware of incremental fluctuations in the body's balance and tension, the student can remain in a relaxed attitude that allows for a proper response. Being able to change with change is to engage. Forcing a situation or being nonresponsive is very stressful.

In the body, tension can be caused by the unnecessary tightening or the dysfunctional releasing of muscles during movement. Grouped as antagonistic pairs, one muscle contracts as another muscle expands to generate flexion and extension. For example, to pull, the biceps contract, while the triceps expand. To push, the triceps contract, while the biceps expand. It is through their mutual cooperation (yinyang) that greater strength, without the loss due to internal restriction, can be produced.

Another source of tension is loss of freedom of movement due to poor joint alignment. If during squatting, the knees are allowed to go past the metatarsals that provide support in the feet, the body's weight no longer goes through the joints into the floor and greater muscular tension (bracing) is required to stabilize the body. Squatting is not as effortless, because the weight bearing joints are now dealing with an added load and cannot flex with ease.

Basically this is a loss of central equilibrium and balance. The weight is shifted forward onto the toes, the heels begin to lift off the floor and are bearing less load, the trunk tips forward trying to balance the body and causes the lower back to seize. This destabilization causes the autonomic nervous system to react to a potential fall by tightening the body further. Relaxation is minimalized.

Tai Chi is the study and practice of "relaxed,

balanced, full body, continuous motion". The mind like a general gives orders to the body and the body acting like a trained army reports back to the mind via body sensations. If the mind does not listen, possibly because it is lost in recalling the choreography, critical information will not be perceived. Thus to reduce tension and increase relaxation, it is imperative to feel your way through the form, rather than force yourself through it. This is relatable to "Use intention, not force" found in Yang Chengfu's Ten Essentials. Use Yi, a clear intention first, then action, not Li, mindless unrestrained brute force. A clear broad perception generates body integration in movement.

As in the case of squatting, the mind's desire is to lower the body down toward the floor. This initiated mental action, will then be followed by a physical reaction. If the mind is only focused on meeting the mental objective, and pays no attention to the moment to moment physical transformations of the body, tension can easily occur due to misalignment and loss of balance. Although through a body awareness (somatic) practice the correct muscles can be utilized, while the corresponding antagonist muscles relax, joints can be rotated into their proper positions, aligned weight distribution can be monitored, and a "path of least resistance" can be sought, relieving tension in movement and amplifying relaxation.

Week 14 – Yinyang

Tai Chi theory is based on the principles of Yinyang interaction. The perfect and complete **Absolute** is comprised of mutually arising interdependent **Relative** opposites. The outer circle represents the wholeness (Tai Chi) of the two combined parts of Yin (black) and Yang (white). The smaller inner circles continue this theory infinitum by illustrating that yin contains yang and yang contains yin. It is important to consider that yin and yang do not represent qualities like superiority and inferiority, good and evil, or love and hate, but seeks to explain the dualistic relations like those that arise between the physical world of the substantial and the insubstantial, the energy of life that is creative and destructive, and the spirit and mind of self and other. Surely without one, the other cannot exist. Yang is categorized as matter, tangible, flesh, male, heavy, hard, day, bright, expanding opening outward, rising upward, advancing, releasing, etc. Yin is categorized as energy, ethereal, spirit, female, light, soft, night, dark, contracting closing inward, descending downward, retreating, storing, etc. When Yang reaches its extreme, it generates Yin and vice versa. This is illustrated at the intersection points found at the top and bottom of the Tai Chi circle. Tai Chi (Grand Extreme) is like the unbroken universal cycles that wax and wane, ebb and flow, and brings dusk back to dawn.

1. Opposition / Contradiction: The principle of opposition can easily be explained in

examining magnetic repulsion. Whereas opposites attract each other (+ to - and - to +), the same polarities repel each other (+ from + and - from -). If an attacker pushes, the defense of pushing back will only be effective if it can overcome the attacker's inertia and applied force by creating a greater force (Force = Mass x Acceleration). This is known as fighting fire with fire, resisting using muscular force rather than yielding like water. Contradiction is addressed in the paradox of the sword and shield. An arms dealer bragged his swords could pierce any shield and his shields could stop any sword. What happens when an unstoppable force meets an immovable object?

2. Interdependence: This is the relationship of relativity. In a three-dimensional reality, center (height) is found in association with length and width.

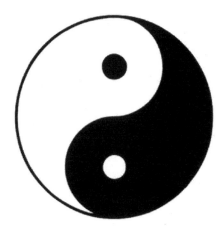

When the body's weight leans forward, the heels may lift, uprooting the back of the base of support. When the body's weight leans back, the balls of the feet may lift, uprooting the front of the base of support. This explains the Tai Chi classic saying, **when you move upward, the mind must be aware of down; when moving forward, the mind also thinks of moving back.** Central equilibrium is constantly maintained by moving from the center (horizontal waist / vertical centerline) and actualizing the relativity of balance and gravity.

3. Mutual Inclusion: Scientifically there is no purity (100%). All distillations will contain some impurity. This is what allows for change through interaction and is illustrated by the two small dots found in the Tai Chi symbol. Yin contains Yang and Yang contains Yin. In empty stepping, the insubstantial leg (Yin) still contains its own mass and possesses the ability to become the substantial leg (Yang) as weight is shifted onto it.

4. Interaction: Due to Interdependence and Mutual Inclusion changing one element affects the other elements. The 5 Directions (center, forward, back, left, right) are an extension of Yinyang theory. A closer examination of shifting forward and back in a bow stance will reveal the centerline travels slightly laterally too. The centerline is closer to the substantial leg. Like any mixture, the proper proportions yield the desired result. If the body is too tight, limp, extended or collapsed the smooth interaction of Yinyang movement is compromised.

5. Complimentary or Mutual Support: In Tai Chi, we yield to the opponent's force, generally following his direction. Then by adding our own energy, we "Push the canoe with the stream". Their energy is supported by our energy. When we use the body propelling both hand in the same direction as in Roll Back, this complimentary energy is described as "Mother - Son". The mother leads and her child follows along energetically. In the west, Tai Chi is expressed as Yin and Yang. This rendering often implies in the mind that they are two separate things. In the east, 陰 陽 translated as one word Yinyang expresses they are interdependent and mutually arising. Philosophically, men (Yang) and woman (Yin) are not superior and subordinate, but equal. Without both, no creation cycle can occur.

6. Change and Transformation: This is the alchemy of Tai Chi. It is our objective in the study and practice of therapeutic exercise that our efforts will produce healthy results. Addressing imbalance in motion will change into a settled, rooted, stable, confident locomotion through a regular practice. Engaging a Somatic "body in mind" awareness brings presence to the mind enhancing mental stability.

The one (Tai Chi as Absolute) creates the Relative two (Yinyang Chaos). These create the three (Yang Zenith, Yin Nadir, Yinyang transformation), This creates the Four Phases of Tai Chi (Extreme Yang, Yang transforming into Yin, Extreme Yin, Yin transforming into Yang). Now the four becomes the Five Elements (Wu Xing). This continues into infinity to create the 10,000 things (alluding to everything).

In addition to its application to the martial arts like Tai Chi Chuan (Boxing), Five Element Theory is also utilized in many other Chinese studies like medicine, music, painting, calligraphy, cooking, religion, geomancy, etc. to further subdivide the Yinyang interplay of Tai Chi transformations. The subject of this paper will express its association to the Five Directions (Center, Front, Back, Left, Right) applied to the Fixed Stepping Method. This method is subdivided into the Five Skills: Shifting, Pivoting, Standing, Stepping, Transitioning.

Shifting changes, the weight distribution on the feet (Base of Support) by moving the Centerline (perineum to crown) while maintaining a vertical alignment (Central Equilibrium). The Centerline is shifted by moving the waist (horizontal alignment) using the legs and feet. Prior to pivoting a foot or lifting a foot for stepping and kicking, weight must be shifted making one leg substantial (supportive) and the other insubstantial (mobilized).

Pivoting rotates the Centerline fixing the foot in the desired direction. It should be noted, after shifting weight off of a leg making it insubstantial and mobilized for pivoting on the heel, the substantial weighted leg maintains the weight throughout the complete pivoting process. Often student erroneously shift their weight back onto the very leg they are trying to pivot effortlessly. The overall objective in movement is to create a Path of Least Resistance and minimizing energy waste by reducing physical restrictions.

Standing supports the entire weight of the body on one leg. To be functional, the substantial leg's hip joint (femur / pelvis) must be able to effortless pivot allowing the insubstantial leg to step without loss of central equilibrium. The upper body must be light, relaxed, and able to move freely. Like a post sunk deep into the ground, the substantial leg and foot roots to the floor.

Stepping (Empty) is an extension of the leg's energy initiated by turning the waist while standing on a substantial leg. Initially, the foot connects to the floor with the heel pad without shifting the weight. Instead of falling onto the heel, the foot immediately provides upward energy supporting the whole body.

Transition After the heel makes contact, the rear leg provides the energy to shift the body forward. The weight distribution on the front foot shifts forward from heel to ball pad (60% ball pad / 40% heel pad). In stepping, the craft is to connect the usage of both legs together into a combined energy through the lower back. Theoretically, **Transition** uses the skill of **Shifting,** but viewed holistically this is the final part of Fixed Stepping were the technique's stored energy is being released, ending one movement and beginning the next.

With practice, the 5 Skills contained in the Fixed Stepping become unified, ultimately returning to the one (Tai Chi). The first two parts (Shift and Pivot) brings the body into the center (Stand), while the final two parts bring the body out of the center (Step and Transition).

The Five Elements are traditionally expressed as cycles (creative example) of Water, Wood, Fire, Earth, Metal...Water. The production of Chi is explained as an alchemy. Wood (fuel) is used to build a Fire on the Earth (ground). A Metal cauldron filled with Water is brought to a boil producing steam (Chi). Steam is refined water with the impurities removed. Analogous to exercise, the body's metabolic processes are stimulated by heightened respiration, circulation, and articulation brought on through movement. The body heats removing impurities through sweat and exhaling. The processes of digestion and elimination are also improved.

In regard to Fixed Stepping, the alchemy can be

explained as "Stand like a mighty mountain (Earth), move like a great river" (Water). Receding backward is like Water yielding. Opening outward is like Wood expanding. Moving forward is like Fire advancing. Standing on one foot is Earth rooting. Closing inward is like Metal condensing. Transitioning continues the cycle (Water). Starting in stillness, a great wave of energy is generated by correctly combining the 5 Elements.

Clarification may be found by viewing the 5 Elements as the 5 Directions (Center, Front, Back, Left, Right). Center is Earth. Front is Yang ascending and moving forward like a Fire. Its Yin complement is Water. Receding (moving back), it descends never failing to reach its lowest level. Metal is Yang (right) and Wood is Yin (left). Like holding a knife in the right hand (moving from outside to in) cutting down rice stalks. The left hand clears (moving inside to out) pushing down the stalks to expose the root. Opening and closing the body are consider functions of Wood (extension / tension) and Metal (flexion / compression). See Tensegrity.

The 5 Skills are whole body functions ultimately unifying into one grand energy.

The 10 Essentials was written by Yang Chengfu (1883 - 1936), the grandson of the founder of Yang Family Tai Chi, Yang Lu Chan. Many translations and explanations have been written to clarify these terse and obscure distillations. In general, it should be taken under consideration that their three main topics of body, energy, and mind, need to be harmonized into an organized whole to reduce flaws and amplify the effectiveness and efficiency of the mind - body in movement.

Number 1: Empty Neck, Raise Spirit

The neck consists of 7 cervical vertebrae. The head is connected to the spine via C1, the first vertebra (Upper Gate). The neck is simply the upper part of the spine. To function properly the spine needs to be aligned and manipulated as a whole. Similar to a snake. When the chin is dropped and the crown raised, the vertebra of the neck open and expand upward with the spine providing ease of movement. This is radically different compared to lifting a pultruding chin and throwing the head back. The vertebra compress and tighten creating impinged restriction.

Conscious awareness is associated with the concept of Spirit. Looking down at the floor or off aimlessly into space, does not direct the intention and collect the spirit as facing something directly. Our outer physical posture is often reflective of how we feel emotionally inside. Feeling down or depressed has an introverted pessimist negativity that traps us inside our intimate personal problems. When the field of consciousness is expanded, usually with the aid of some form of mind / body therapy, it begins to dissolve this self-imposed separation between inner and outer space, generating a cathartic feeling of hope and possible resolution. This positive optimism is fundamental to healing and improvement. Looking to the brighter side (outside the body), chin up, and pull yourself up by your own bootstraps (self-empowerment) are all analogous to raising the spirit.

Energy is rooted in the Earth (solid) mainly through the ball pads of the feet, transferred through the body (made mostly of formless Water), and because we stand upright, we have an intangible connection to Heaven (Gas / atmosphere) with the crown of our head. When we inhale air, the diaphragm descends and the spine expands upward, providing a feeling of leading energy up the back. When we exhale waste, the diaphragm ascends and the spine contracts, providing a feeling of leading energy down the front. Between the eyebrows is the third eye. This is known as the upper Dan Tien where the Spirit (Shen) resides. Mind (Xin) is the heart / mind. The proper combination of the mind's Intention (Yi) and the body's emotional sensation, creates a unified spirit encompassing both mind and body.

Week 17 – Essential 2

Number 2: Contain Chest, Raise Back

Now that the head has been discussed in relation to the spine, the middle area (ribcage) needs to be clarified. When the chest is contained (collar bones low) and not braced upward, which causes the shoulder blades to pinch together, the arms can open laterally via the back without impingement and move freely dimensionally. The interconnectedness of torso and arms takes place as the chest (anterior) relaxes down and the upper back (posterior), in association with the spine, moves vertically upward. When the back (spine) is compressed, the shoulders moved backwards, and the lower back severely curved inward, a swayed back posture results. Although self-help movement practices can be therapeutic, some deeper postural abnormalities need professional medical intervention.

The shoulder blades work with the elbows to connect the arms to the spine. Vertebra T2 and T3 (Middle Gate) located in the upper back need to move freely to acquire this freedom and range of movement. The combination of horizontal arms and a vertical spine forms a plus sign (+) configuration of the body. Actualizing the function of their intersection is key by simultaneously containing the chest and raising the back. This body unification is known as the Power of Ten because the Chinese character for ten is written as +. Engaging this relationship fortifies three-dimensional movement and energy generation.

The phrase "round the back" like a turtle shell helps to express a feeling of creating a ring around the body. The arms are unified together through the back. Connecting the arms to the spine is essential to full body usage in movement. The Middle Gate, shoulder blades, shoulders, elbows, wrists, and middle fingers form an external ring around the outside of the arms. A complimentary ring runs inside the arms across the chest associated with the Middle Dan Tien (Solar Plexus / Heart).

It is important to remember there are no fixed postures. Statically or dynamically there are always internal processes taking place in the torso continuously. In regard to the thoracic cavity, the ceaseless respiration via the lungs and the circulation of blood via the heart benefits greatly from reduced internal muscular tension and physical restriction. Working in proper conjunction with the abdomen and the lower back (Lower Gate), the diaphragm can be provided ample room to descend and ascend with less impingement improving lung function.

We do not want to force movement or breathing, but instead remove the restrictions to ease of movement which in turn will strengthen our stability and deepen our relaxation. Evoking softness is the methodology.

Number 3: Loosen Waist

The body is divided into three sections: upper, middle, and lower. The waist is the middle that connects above and below. The coordination of the arms and legs to create whole body usage is controlled and directed by the waist movements. When the waist is relaxed, there is body connection. When the waist tightens, separation occurs resulting in compartmental use of individual body parts instead of a cohesive whole.

The lower back, vertebrae L2 and L3 form the Lower Gate. Working with the crotch area in the front known as the Kua, the pelvic is able to swing freely like a hammock supported between two trees (legs). Done in a dynamic fashion this is known as a pelvic thrust. Although in regard to spinal alignment used in movement, properly dropping the lower back and rounding the Kua, opens and straighten the 5 lumbar vertebrae facilitating better connection between waist and the lower body (legs and feet). When turning the waist on one leg, the hip is the connection between the pelvis and the upper thigh bone that is used as a pivot point in stepping.

While in a Bow stance, the waist leads the energy stored in the legs to **shift the weight** distribution between the legs. In a forward Bow stance, the front leg is flexed, substantially storing a potential to move backward. Here the hip connection via the knee and ankle finds an energetic root to the Earth via the foot. Often is the case, the other insubstantial rear leg's hip connection is not receptive to the backward movement. The leg should be straight but not locked at the knee. Thinking of the two legs working as one through the waist (Ming Men: Lower Gate T2 / T3) is a good practice to make the legs more functional in usage. The Kua should be rounded like the arch in a bridge. When the center of gravity is too high, the legs form a triangular teepee shape configuration which locks up the hip connection reducing waist freedom. Song: sinking and relaxing is essential.

Additional range of motion can be found in **rotating the centerline**. Instead of the hip facilitating movement, the waist's connective tissue above the hip, rotates the center line left and right tuning the torso horizontally. This is like the Earth's rotation on its axis. Lower back kidney area muscles are utilized.

Keeping the middle area pliant allows for full dimensional movement. Exploring the waist's relevance to pivoting the waist, shifting the weight, and rotating the centerline will further the actualization of whole body usage.

Number 4: Differentiate Empty Full

This is often described as "distinguish substantial (full) and insubstantial (empty)". It is the application of Yinyang theory. Initially students often think of this only in terms of weight distribution. While standing entirely on one leg, it is full of the body's weight and the other is completely empty of all weight. Although this is not an incorrect perception, thinking in terms of the potential of energy is more consistent with the practice of movement; "continuous motion without interruption". The full leg has the potential (stored energy) not only to bear the entire body's weight, but also to energize the waist rotation needed to initiate the empty leg's step. Once the empty leg's foot makes contact with the ground via the Empty Step Method, the full leg's potential can be released shifting the body.

Regarding the body, in Empty Stepping also known as Yinyang Stepping, the weight is either 100% on the right leg (yang) or the left leg (yin). The transitions between these two extremes are Yang going yin and yin going yang. At some point in the transition, the weight is distributed 50% on each leg (double weighted).

Regarding the potential (energy), the leg that bears 100% of the weight (full) has stored energy (yang). The other leg is empty (yin) and has the potential to receive and store energy when the full leg releases its potential. In studying Tai Chi theory, it is important to first establish the category of discussion (body, energy, etc.) prior to determining the Yinyang relationships.

The legs are unified through the waist. Mainly the lower gate in the back (Ming Men L2 / L3) and the Kua (crotch) in the front. The Centerline (perineum to crown) is moved by the waist. The waist directs the motion of the body by using the energy potential exchanged in the legs.

Standing on one leg (full), **Collect** the energy. Stepping with the other leg (empty) and touching the floor (forward use heel pad or backward use ball pad) with no weight is **Connect**. Without pause or falling (forward or backward) into the ground, immediate support is sought as the body is shifted. This is **Transfer** the energy.

The object of differentiating empty full is to ultimately unify the whole body into one effective and efficient energy (Tai Chi). Studying and clarifying the parts (Yinyang) in the mind, forms the intention of the body practice. The ability to feel through sensation; balance, stability, relaxation, ease of movement, integrated movement, emotional serenity, etc. is the means to obtaining a Tai Chi (Yinyang) body.

Number 5: Sink Shoulders, Drop Elbows

The arms connect energetically to the spine at the Middle Gate located at T2/T3. This connection can be functionally felt as the shoulder blades are moved away laterally from the spine, moving the elbows left and right. Essential 2: Contain Chest, Raise Back is fundamental to this articulation.

Dropping the elbows downward allows the rotator cuffs to align and function properly without impingement. When the arms are raised and the shoulders are erroneously lifted as in shrugging, the elbows lift, restricting the rotator cuffs, the neck tightens (C1 compresses), and the shoulder blades are pulled in toward the spine limiting freedom of movement and whole body usage.

Instead of the upper body muscles being relaxed and the torso weight dropping down (Song) into the legs, this unnecessary tightness caused by incorrectly raising the Chi (energizing muscles), is the source of loss of ease of movement and range of movement in the arms. The upper body should be at ease and light.

Often this problem occurs in stepping, especially when standing and pivoting on one legs. The upper body is erroneously braced by contracting muscles in an attempt to create and maintain stability.

It is imperative to clearly understand that the spine is made of 24 independent vertebrae. A malfunction in alignment in one area will often cause a restriction in another area. Think of the Spine (viewed from the posterior) as a slightly convex bow. Viewing the perineum and crown as the ends, the Three Gates: L2/L3, T2/T3, and C1 act as the main focal points for aligning all 24 vertebra of the spine in motion.

In this respect, the functional alignment of the three joints of the arms; shoulder, elbow, and wrist in movement must be considered too. Ultimately, our study focuses on the objective of whole body usage in movement. Misaligning, locking, and impinging one joint usually negatively affects the one above and the one below.

The energy of Push can be used as a means to improve shoulder and elbow flexion and extension. When retracting the arms, the rotator cuffs in the shoulders rotate back and down and the elbows are dropped down toward the floor. As the arms extend, the cuffs rotate forward and up (the energy comes up for under the armpits) and the elbows should not lock. Lock the elbows and notice how it lifts the shoulders and affects the upper back creating tension in the lower back too. To take advantage of whole body energy, applying all 10 Essentials is key.

Number 6: Use Intention, not Exertion

This is commonly stated as Use Intention 意 not Force 力. Intention (Yi) is an idea or expectation that is generated in the mind. The stronger and clearer this mental directive is, a greater control over the Xing 形 (body, shape, form) usage is obtained. This can be considered as the mental scholarly / academic knowledge that is verified to be effective and efficient through an in depth physical body practice. Metaphorically it is to possess a key that easily opens a door.

Force (Li) is power and strength. Here it is being expressed not as the application of a refined energy, but as a crude and wasteful form of overexertion. Metaphorically, instead of searching for the key to open a door, unbridled force is applied relentlessly until it is busted down. Like using a sledgehammer to kill a mosquito. In Tai Chi, the study and practice is to use softness to overcome hardness, the internal to control the external, and expressed as mind over matter.

Sir Isaac Newton's Third Law of Motion states, "For every action, there is an equal and opposite reaction". While shifting forward in a bow stance, the rear leg's extension creates a force that moves the body forward. The front leg's improper flexion can create a greater resistance to this movement by poor balance (loss of central equilibrium), misaligned joints, and unnecessary muscular tension. Ease of movement is reduced and a greater force must be generated by the rear leg to overcome these self-generated impingements. It is through a slow and soft incremental movement practice that the body can be studied. The mind's blindness to the body's articulation is usually the source of excessive force and wasted energy.

Inertia and continuous motion / movement (Review Newton's first and second laws of motion) are components of generating force. Force is equal to mass times acceleration ($F = M \times A$). In form practice, being continuously in control through the application of intentional incremental energy is preferable to loss of control through the generation of a free falling momentum, comparable to a snowball rolling uncontrollably down a hill. Accelerating the body (mass) is directed by the waist, controlling the energy developed in the legs and initiated by the root. (feet on the floor).

By realizing the flaws in movement and actualizing refined body usage, the mind's intention becomes the driving force of the body. Matter and energy are the same. Essentially, the mind (Yi) leads the energy (Chi) throughout the body, creating the muscular contractions of articulation that generates the force (Li) expressed by the arms and hands. The mind is the body. The body is the mind.

Number 7: Upper Lower Mutually Follow

Often this is rendered as Upper Body and Lower Body Work Together. In practical application, the objective is to unify the energy of the whole body to create a single directional force. For study purposes, the body is divided into upper, middle (waist), and lower. The 6 External Harmonies is used to comprehend the synchronization of the flexing and extending action of the arm (upper) and leg (lower) joints under the direction of the waist.

The hip / shoulder joints, knee / elbow joints, and ankle / wrist joints are paired together. Considering there are two arms and two legs, the flexing and extending of the joints, leading to the opening and closing the body, can take on many variations depending on the specific energy being created. Examining push and pull is a good place to start this study.

Push - From a left foot forward bow stance, shifting back, the right leg is flexed storing energy. At the same time, the right arm is flexed creating the potential to release the energy of push. In execution, the right leg and right arm will extend under the direction of the waist movement coordinating together to emit the power.

Pull - From a left foot forward bow stance, the left leg is flexed storing energy. At the same time, the right arm is extended creating the potential to release the energy of pull. In execution, the left leg extends, the waist turns right, and the right arm flexes, coordinating together to generate power unified by the waist.

In light of this clarification, it is easy to understand the energy is rooted in the foot. Developed by the leg (hip, knee, ankle). Directed by the waist. Expressed by the arm (shoulder, elbow, wrist) and hand.

This essential is about coordinating the action of the arms and legs together to create power. It is implied there is an understanding that loss of central equilibrium, improper joint alignment, and unnecessary muscular tension are flaws that are detrimental to this process. A common fault is instead of directing from the waist and unifying upper and lower, the Tai Chi movements are led by the hands.

When the form is performed without skills like those found in the 10 Essentials, externally there is movement, but internally no functional energies are developed. Movements generate the potential to actualize the 8 Energies of Tai Chi. The intentionally soft, slow, incremental practice of the form is to improve function. Without the mind's illumination of the essential in practice, the body is a rudderless boat.

Number 8: Inner Outer Mutually Harmonize.

The "conscious" mind receives information as five "objects of perception" (form, sound, smell, taste, physical sensation) separately from each of the five "organs of perception" (eye, ear, nose, tongue, body). Although, the mind does perceive reality raw and simple, it uses discrimination and the emotions to form a personal biased perspective (opinion). This subjective view is further enhanced by considering the objective view of others and the impossibility to know all.

The interdependence of the mind and body (yinyang) is brought into unification (Taiji) through study and practice. "Embody the yin and embrace the yang", expresses the mind is externalized into the body. Gathering and taking in information to express it outward functionally.

Yin is the Mother of Yang. Energy originates as yin; bottom to top, inside to out, back to front. Rooted feet, energetic hands. Respiration and blood circulation, muscles express the energy. The past action influences the present moment.

Internally during inhalation, feel the body open and expand externally. Mentally, relax the body to further the body's opening. Both the mind and the body open together. Externally during exhalation, feel the body close and contract. Perceiving inside the body using the mind's eye and experiencing the sensation, embody this contraction. Be the movement with the whole body and mind.

This is the essence of internal training. The internal mind's eye perceives and directs the body's action. Later once refined skills have been obtained, the attention and action can be externalized to engage the world and respond to conditions. A trained mind perceives what is important and does not get attached to emotional states. Essential 9 "Continuous motion without interruption" pertains not only to the body, but also when the mind stops and becomes disconnected to the present body action. It is very challenging in meditation to keep the mind from wandering off and entertaining irrelevant ideas as the body goes off on a journey of rote recitation.

The present opens a gate to a vast and open field. Our past experiences and our future aspirations can be either advantageous or destructive to our goals. It is in the present moment where the mind and body have the opportunity to actualize our goal. The change that we seek happens now. Harmonizing inner and outer requires a resolution of both mind and body. Fear in the mind is expressed in the body. Strength in the body can fortify the mind. When mind and body are truly one, the unification of Taiji (Yinyang) is actualized. Free and fully awake.

Number 9: Linked without Interruption

Tai Chi Chuan is known as Long Fist which is comparable to the ocean's waves, where its energy is unified (a body of water), continuous, and without beginning or end. Unlike generating a crude external force, where a person struggles to raise its required energy, fights to connect to its natural flow, and continues till it is fully exhausted, internal energy does not end in one direction until it gives rise to a potential of reversal. The whole body and mind is constantly employed.

For example, when shifting forward into a bow stance, the back leg is "straight, but not straight" and the front leg is "curved, but not curved". If the back leg completely extends; straightening and locking the hip, knee and ankle joints, the leg loses its functional potential to flex and move the body backward. If the front leg's flexes too much; closing and tightening, it loses its functional potential to extend the joints and move the body backward. The movement is no longer cyclical, but stop and go linear. A greater force must be generated to overcome these self-generated impingements and restrictions to ease of movement. The Chi of the body is disconnected and the body become compartmentalized in movement.

When this Essential is translated as "Movement without Interruption", it is often misunderstood as only the external body must keep moving.

Although this is true visually, it is the unseen internal effectiveness of the body's correct usage in movement that is of greater value. Movement is linked together by the individual skills (gong) that creates the various movements found in the form. Shifting generates Pivoting. Pivoting generates Standing. Standing generates Empty Stepping. Empty Stepping generates Transitioning. These Five Skills are linked together by continuous waist usage.

A traditional expression is "Dragon head, Snake tail. It warns of starting with robust mental and physical energy and ending drained. The energy should be consistent, so it has the potential to continue. Often students begin a twenty-five-minute practice of the 103 Long Form with an attitude of mental concentration and physical clarity, only to speed up and rush to finish. To this end, a practice session is for the body, energy, and mind. The mind's clarity of intention, calm demeanor, and attention to detail leads the energy through the body, that in turn articulates the body.

Fundamental to proper practice is that the moments are internally generated in the mind and externalized through the body. "Imagination becomes reality" is to attain an unbroken communication between the physical and mental realms of reality.

Number 10: Move from Center, Seek calm

Also written, seek the tranquility in movement; stillness in motion and motion in stillness. This apparent paradox is actualized as equanimity; maintaining calm and harmonizing with the continuous flux of nature. Everything is in a constant state of change. Yin generates the egg and receives the seed that gives birth to Yang. Yang generates the seed that fertilizes the egg of Yin and receives life from Yin. Together they perpetuate a continuous cycle whose interconnection is essential to the creative and destructive cycles of existence and nonexistence.

Tai Chi as a study seeks to overcome hardness with softness and overcome motion with stillness. Envision a wheel on a fixed axle. Viewed as a functional whole, the wheel moves feely around an immoveable center. Also comparable to a hurricane or whirlpool where the vortex swirls around a calm center. Holistically, one part is still, the other in motion. Viewed from a calm center, the arms and legs orbit around like the planets around the Sun. Orderly, measured, and predictable.

"As above, so below. As within, so without. As the universe, so the soul." is a statement acknowledging that the celestial order is mirrored here on Earth. Taken further, the macrocosmic of the universe in contained inside the human body as the microcosmic. Finding your physical, energetic, and spiritual centers, guarding, and cultivating them is the path to extending yourself into the world. If you are not in control, the forces of nature and other people will take control of your life.

Through a physical body practice we have the opportunity to learn to deal with these external forces, by first addressing our inner responses to our own decisions and actions. For example, in stepping, kicking, and pivoting on a single foot, the body's weight must be continuously managed to prevent loss of balance and falling. Shifting uses the rooted feet and legs / the waist directs the centerline adjusting the weight distribution and energy potential / the centerline closer to one leg properly, results in one leg supporting like a mountain, while the other leg flows like a river. Gravity is always at work. Aligning with it is the practice.

Initially, students struggle with themselves. Balance is tenuous. Insubstantial. The Five Skills are not clear individually or linked smoothly together. How Yinyang movement and stillness are interdependent is a mystery. Tranquility is an unbroken thread like a body of water that rises and falls, ebbs and flows. The steady consistency of calm stillness is blended with the ever changing dynamics of movement. In motion, Tai Chi combines. The two become one. In stillness, Tai Chi separates. The one become two. We are both actor and audience. Subject and object.

Week 26 - Lower Gate

Name: Ming-men / Gate of Life

Location: L2 / L3 (GV - 4)

Function:

Physically this Gate energetically connects the pelvic area to the torso.

This area of the spine has a natural curvature that can be manipulated by a movement similar, but not as dynamic to a pelvic thrust. Here the pelvic is rolled under slightly, lowing the coccyx, so the perineum is on the bottom pointing toward the floor. This results in a straightening of the lower vertebrae. It should be noted, that the pelvis is not rolled in the opposite direction past the spine's natural concave curvature. This results in an undesirable compression of the lower vertebra. Naturally this Gate is always half closed / half open. Manipulating this gate acts like a pump, further increasing the movement of energy in the body. Up the back, down the front.

Energetically this Gate connects the Jing (Essence stored in kidneys) with the Chi (Intrinsic Energy) stored in the solar plexus area.

This process of internal alchemy can simply be understood as; consumed food and water is processed in the stomach and intestine, combines with the oxygen via the lungs is circulated by the blood through the pumping action of the heart, delivering these essential nutrients throughout the entire body. The resulting cumulative action manifests itself as Reproductive Energy (Jing - Essence), Chi (Intrinsic Energy), and Shen (the illumination of the Heart / Mind).

This gate is referenced in Essential # 2 Loosen Waist. Raising the lower back amplifies the natural curve compressing the vertebrae and causing the chest to lift forward impinging the shoulder blades of the arms. It is important to remember that a change in one area of the spine is reflected in another area of the spine.

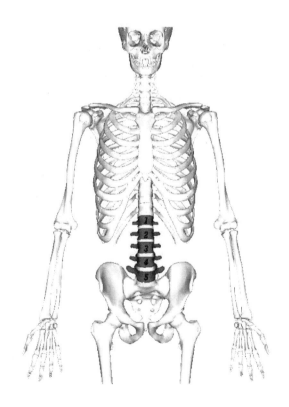

Week 27 - Middle Gate

Location: T2 / T3

The spine governs up and down. The arms across the back governs left and right.

This Gate is the point of intersection. "Contain chest, raise (upper) back" is a vertical function. (Do not pin the shoulder blades together, impinging the arms)

"Sink shoulders, drop elbows" creates functional rotation. Do not impinge the free articulation of the arms via the rotator cuff.

Moving the shoulder blades is a lateral - left and right function. (Do not pull the arms behind the body) "Opening and closing the body" begins on the inside.

The body contains 5 Bows comprised of the 9 Gates.

The spine (L2/L3, T2/T3, C1), the two arms (shoulder, elbow, wrist), and the two legs (hip, knee, ankle). Correct directional alignment is critical to functional movement.

Just like a conventional bow and arrow, they close flexing in one direction and open extending in the other direction. Movement stores and releases energy.

The both arms as a unit and both legs as another unit, can be considered as greater bows, with the "center" of the bows located at the Spine. The lower gate connects the legs together like a keystone of an arch bridge. The middle gate functions like a crossroad. Energy up the spine is directed into the arm via this gate.

Character Ten Power

The Chinese character for the number ten looks like a plus sign. (+) The muscles that power the arms for lifting, lowering, pushing, and pulling are in the back and chest. The training objective is to attain a holistic harmony of total body usage in movement and reduce the flaw of compartmental usage of singular parts of the body.

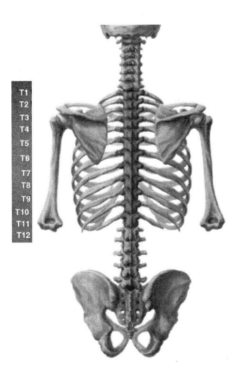

Week 28 - Upper Gate

Location: C1

There are 7 cervical vertebrae. C1 is on the top under the skull.

The head requires support from a straight and expanded (open) neck.

Slightly lowering the chin and drawing it in, will make C1 act like a hinge, opening and closing this gate. Erroneously lifting the face and pushing the head forward, places the head in front of the body, providing poor support and seizing the neck.

As with the manipulation of all the gates, fixed stiff positions are never the objective. When all 3 Gates are actively engaged, the spine as a whole can expand upward (Yang Chengfu's 10 Essentials # 1) raising a light, lively, and intangible energy to the top of the head. If the gates are not properly aligned, to open the spine undue force is required to push through restriction, resulting in increased muscular tension and weakening the root (foot connection to the ground). The spine elongates from the bottom up. The head feels suspended from above.

The lower body is heavy like a Jade Table because it is always under the compression of the upper body weight. Properly supported continuously by the lower body (waist and legs) the upper body can remain light, relaxed, and supple throughout the movements. The middle body (waist) is loose and can move freely like a Lazy Susan.

When manipulating the 3 Gates in the back it is important to consider their associated areas in the front.

Lower Gate Drop lower back, round Kua

Middle Gate Raise (upper) back, contain chest

Upper Gate Empty neck, lower chin

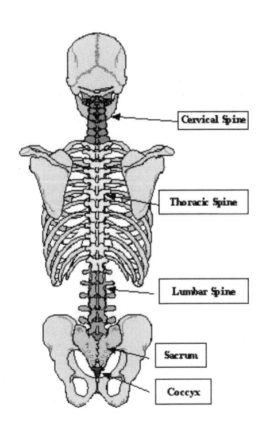

Cervical Spine

Thoracic Spine

Lumbar Spine

Sacrum

Coccyx

Week 29 – Breathing 1

Diaphragmatic Breathing - Abdominal / Belly

The core of 氣 功 Qigong is breathing exercises. Although applicable, it differs from robust physical calisthenics like aerobics and résistance training, where the accelerated body movements and added load causes the lungs to increase respiration, thus fulfilling the body's need for more oxygen by increasing blood circulation with a faster heartbeat.

Qigong begins as a static body study how to breath more effectively and efficiently by examining the mechanics of breathing. Cerebral knowledge is combined with physical sensation experienced in practice. Relaxation is essential. Consistent patient effort is paramount.

In & Out
The objective is not to force more air in, but to reduce the restrictions usually caused by incorrect joint alignment and poor body usage. The diaphragm is a muscle located underneath the lungs that is drawn down, descending towards the intestine during inhalation. During exhalation, the diaphragm is released rising upward, moving the air out of the lungs. Nasal respiration is preferred, but mouth exhalation is also used to remove heat.

Open & Close
In articulating the arms and legs in movement, opening and closing is defined as moving the limbs away from the torso (centerline), but this process actually starts internally and radiates outward coordinated with the breathing process. As the diaphragm descends during inhalation, allowing the lower abdomen to expand outward unrestricted (open), removes a major blockage to the diaphragm's downward expansion. When the abdomen distends, it allows the internal

organs to move away freely from the descending diaphragm, removing restriction to its movement. This creates a softer easier fuller air intake. As the diaphragm ascends during exhalation, the abdomen contracts (close) correctly.

In typical Yinyang fashion, addressing the abdomen in the front, the Lower Gate (命 門 Ming Men) in the back can remove restriction too. "Dropping the Back" and opening this energy gate in the spine (L2 / L3) alleviates abdominal restrictions to the diaphragm's movement. Remember to open and round the crotch (Kua) when articulating the Lower Gate.

In Part 2, the upper chest and ribcage associated with thoracic breathing which is integral to diaphragmatic breathing, will be discussed. It is the integration of the whole body that leads to a greater achievement. Always reference a global perspective of the body when refining individual parts. Don't miss the forest for the trees.

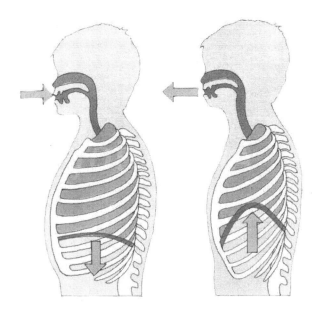

Week 30 – Breathing 2

Diaphragmatic Breathing - Thoracic / Chest

To be clear. Regardless if you are just performing the lower abdominal breathing or adding the upper thoracic breathing by filling and broadening the chest laterally, the alignment of the whole spine is always important. In breathing, in addition to the previous mentioned In & Out and Open & Close, the spine needs to extend and flex vertically; Up & Down as the lungs expand and contract throughout the respiratory process. The correct coordinated articulation of the arms aids the thoracic breath by helping to open the torso.

Starting in the Prepare Stance with the arms relaxed down and the palms facing the abdomen, Exhale. Beginning with the left drawing below, abdominally inhale as the arms coil laterally and slightly forward, palms facing front. Feel the Lower Gate opening. Continue with the thoracic breath as the arms ascend laterally, opening the middle gate and expanding the shoulder blades. The hands arc about the level of the solar plexus. As the breathing continues, arms raising above the head, feel the upper gate open by expanding the neck, and finish with the palms facing down pointed toward the crown of the head. Essentially, the spine needs to extend as the lungs fills with air. While exhaling, lower both hands down the front of the body on each side of the centerline, palms facing in. Basically both arms are performing downward circles. Feel the spine close and flex. Imagine energy ascending up the back during inhalation and descending down the front during exhalation.

When the spine fails to open correctly, not only is respiration restricted, but instead of the feet staying flat and rooted to the Earth, the body is pulled upward by the lifting action of the arms and balance is compromised. It is important to remember, the body is not forced open by applying excessive muscle, but by removing restrictions from the path of movement and creating a relaxed greater range of motion. After the proper body alignments in motion are thoroughly actualized, it is the subtle breath that can be used to move the body. The body feels far less mechanical because motion is experienced as if the breath is leading the movement. The mind moves the energy and the energy moves the body. Moment by moment and increment by increment. Slow, soft, mentally absorbed movement.

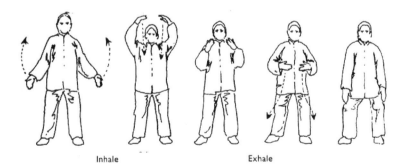

Inhale   Exhale

Week 31 – Breathing 3

Diaphragmatic Breathing and Meditation

The inhalation only needs to fill the lungs to 80 percent capacity. If excessive tension is created during respiration it will be detrimental to the free movement of the body. Internal capacity will increase slowly over time through the yielding action of the body. Never force the breath in. Instead relax deeper to allow the body to expand further. Aspire to a silent, soft, slow, deep, and long respiration.

The exhalation only needs to empty the lungs 80 percent. The inhale and exhale should not feel rushed, sharp, and linear, but rather like a smooth transition, gentle and curved. Breathing is cyclical. The objective is to restore the natural breath to full functionality. Lead the action with your mind. Experience, don't anticipate.

The mind leads the breath. By inducing deep physical relaxation and removing internal restrictions to respiration, the breath naturally slows and becomes effortless. This type of breathing acts as a form of meditation that places the mind into a state that is conducive to healing and stress reduction. Past and future events are replaced with the present. External reality is replaced with the internal landscape of the body. Don't force the breath into an idealized concept of perfection.

Lowering the eyelids so they are only a quarter open, directs the intention inside, but not so far as to completely lose all external reality. The outside of the body can be observed in the light of day, but the inside of the body is dark and mysterious to the eye. Internal vision requires using sensation and the mind's illumination of the body anatomy.

Just like it is possible to interpret the arcane

symbols making up the alphabet into words which create vivid images in the mind, the same imagination can make breathing meditation into an experience that is difficult to fully describe accurately. The body's energy (Chi) becomes vivid and manageable. A feeling of connectedness and wholeness brings a sense of peace, security, and autonomy.

Regardless if lying down, sitting, or standing, breathing is the gateway that connects the mind and body. The lower abdomen becomes the focal point of respiration. In Qigong it is known as the lower Dan Tian. Dan is medicine and Tian is the field where it is cultivated. Usually the mind's attention resides in the head, often deep in thought or lost in a wandering array of discursive agitations. Focusing on the breathing action seeks to strengthen mind body unification.

Once the mind can harness the ocean of energy found in the lower Dan Tian it is possible to direct its energy throughout the body. Initially students focus on the torso; up the back during inhalation and down the front during exhalation. This is known as the Microcosmic Orbit. Once the energy is felt streaming in these two channels, the arms and legs are added. This is known as the Grand Circulation.

The study and practice of Tai Chi Chuan is based on the Method. The Method is the application of the theories and principles of Tai Chi (Yinyang). Tai Chi (Interdependent complementary opposites) exercises strengthen a practitioner's Center and the actualization of balancing Yinyang energies in movement. The "continuous without interruption" movements of the Tai Chi Form are fortified by a One Pointed mentality in the midst of the physical stillness, found in the Post Standing (Zhan Zhuang) exercises.

Often used in external martial arts as a muscular form of endurance testing, the true purpose is an internal struggle to make fine adjustments to the physical structure (alleviating tension by opening blockages), mentally induce deep relaxation, sink into the root (Song), feel the internal movement of energy (Chi) via breathing methods, and improve mental intention (direct spontaneity).

Two basic methods.
Yin - A taller stance, due to its ease of position, allows the practitioner to concentrate easier on the internal movement of Chi via the breathing methods. Holding the arms up, require additional attention to proper structure, so the position acts as an asset to breathing and does not create energetic blockages.

Yang - After gaining proficiency in the Yin method, this method is practiced. The (light) upper body is placed on top of a (heavy) lower body. Obviously the leg muscles will be engaged more dynamically by lowering the center of gravity. The objective is to keep the upper body free of tension (Sink the Chi to the Dan Tien), so it can breathe freely, supplying additional energy to the lower "seated" body.

It cannot be stressed enough that this is a practice of Mind Over Matter (Use Intention, Not Force). It is an intellectual study of physical structure, breathing, and mental visualizations.

Like discovering a key to unlock a door, minimal force is required to enter into the treasure house. Making the best of a tough situation develops character and fortitude. Searching for a solution brings insight. The mind and body unify in this active inactivity meditation.

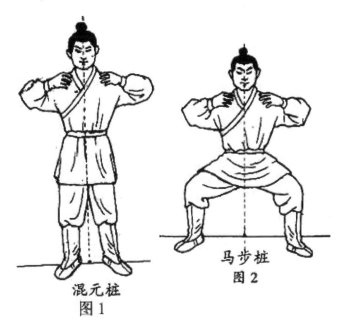

混元桩
图 1

马步桩
图 2

Secret is written in Chinese uses two characters: 秘 secret, mysterious, abstruse and 密 dense, thick, close, intimate. In the martial arts, the connotation is that the knowledge may be easily taught, but it is only through kung fu (effort and time) training that the true potential can be discovered internally and expressed externally by the student. It is often stated in kung fu circles, "There are no secrets".

The Fusion of the Five Elements is an extension of Taiji theory. When the parts are transmuted they form a cohesive whole. Like a chain, strength lies in attending to the weakest link.

Root to the Earth: Earth is the Mother of the Five Elements. The body's center of gravity (waist / lower Dan Tian) finds greater stability lowered downward closer toward the Earth. The Center like an ocean of stored energy (Hara), developed by the legs and rooted by the feet, draws energy up from the ground. The stillness and supportive dependability of the ground (Earth) is the root of movement.

Expand Upward: Fire naturally rises and spreads dimensionally. This open expansion (Fun kai) allows the joints to articulate freely. It counter balances the compression of weight. Although, over expansion can destroy balance by severing the root.

Deep Relaxation: Water naturally recedes back and down seeking the lowest level. Deep relaxation (song) sinks the body's upper energies back down to the lower Dan Tian for storage and utilization. The lower abdomen houses the majority of the body's liquids. Like ballast in a ship, it stabilizes the body. Tension restricts movement and wastes energy. Relaxed abdominal breathing gathers energy internally.

Express Energy Outward: Wood is rooted in the Earth and grows upward toward Heaven. Like a tree, its branches (arms and legs) radiate outward from the trunk (centerline). Opening the body; moving the arms (sequentially shoulder, elbow, wrist) and legs (sequentially hip, knee, ankle) away from the spine, sends energy outward from the Center. Don't lead and pull with the hands and feet.

One Point Concentration: Metal as a mineral ore is produced deep under pressure in the Earth. Where wood extends outward, metal contracts inward. Closing the arms and legs inward toward the center (Yin) is directly related to the function of outwardly opening the limbs (Yang). It is said, Wood is like clearing a field. Pushing down the stalks; in to out (extending) preparing to cut them down at the root, and Metal is like the cleaving ax moving from out to in (contracting). Together they form the basis of blocking out and striking in. Metal destroying wood.

The first phase of study and practice is **physical**. Here the choreography is thoroughly memorized and is used as a venue to understand the advantageous nature of correct joint rotation and alignment to improving ease and range of movement. Functional balance improves as the student learns to move from the waist and maintain central equilibrium consistently. The second phase concerns the **energy** of the body. Breathing exercises are essential to developing a feeling of internal expansion and contraction inside the torso. Directly experiencing and working with the rising and falling physical sensations (tightness, looseness, instability, heaviness, lightness, etc.) generated in movement is a key element of this exploration. The third phase is the **spiritual / mental** development. Learning to "lead the movement with the mind" moment by moment, increment by increment with a clearer intention is the practice. Letting go of discursive thoughts while meditating and focusing the mind with "one-point concentration" develops the power of presence.

Internal practice is to train these three treasures of the body from ordinary levels into the extraordinary realm. They always function as a whole, but studying them individually is a methodology to attain their greater unification. A gestalt.

Yin is the Mother of Yang. The mind can enhance body usage and energy movement by applying these three studies. The mind leads the Qi. Qi leads the body.

Qi moves from bottom to top

Like the roots of a tree, the feet on the ground are the foundation of everything that exists above. Any movement like stepping, kicking, extending the arms, etc. that severs this Earthly connection weakens the energy moving up the body creating the movement. This emphasizes the critical requirement of "functional" balance.

The feet are the body's base of support. The legs provide an upward energy supporting the body like a heavy jade table. The center of gravity; waist must remain loose and free to rotate. The upper body is light and articulate.

Push example: Assume a front stance. Shift the weight back storing energy in the rear leg. Raise the energy up through the back foot that is rooted to the ground, direct the energy through the three gates of the extending back leg (ankle, knee, hip), through the waist, up through the two gates of the spine (lower L2/L3 and middle T2/T3), into the three gates of the arms (shoulder, elbow, wrist) and out the palms. This exercise leads the energy through the body. As the body is moving, the mind directs its intention through the path of energy found in the body. Body sensations and mental awareness work together to refine the articulation of the body.

Qi cultivates internally and radiates externally

In order of priority; oxygen, water, and food are the basic requirements taken internally to sustain life. Qigong includes the study of the breath of life and maintaining its natural order through blood circulation via the arteries and veins to all points in the body. Practice is to alleviate internal structural blockages and restrictions caused by unnecessary muscular tension, misaligned joints, and negative emotional states that impede the radiance of health.

Qi is a synergistic result of various bodily functions coming together to produce vitality and health. Broadening awareness by the absorption of knowledge, enlightens the mind and leads to advantageous physical actions. Ignorance as indifference is often counterproductive to the generation of the life force.

Kick example: Aware of sensation, mentally lead the Qi from the bottom; up and out. Raise the energy up from the rooted foot, through the 3 leg gates of the supporting leg and 3 spine gates*. Direct the energy out the lower gate and through the 3 leg gates of the kicking leg, while simultaneously sending energy out the middle gate and down both 3 arm gates opening the cross hands. *Even though C1 is not in the direct path of energy expression, its correct alignment is essential too.

Qi moves from back (past) to front (future)

According to alchemy theory, opening the three gates in the back, fosters Qi movement up the back and down the front filling the three Dan Tian by utilizing an improved energy circulation method known as the Microcosmic Orbit.

In the martial arts to attack forward, the Qi is rooted in the back foot, developed in the back leg, and sent through the entire body to the hand as the front leg offers greater support and stores an energy potential to move the body backward.

Time ceaselessly slips into the future.
Opportunity is easily lost.
Tonight, all of our lives are decreased by one day.
Heed this warning.
Do not squander your life.

Walking example: It is the back foot root that propels the body forward. Our past actions condition the future. Keep to the center and pay close attention to developing events, instead of losing focus while lost in thoughts of expected results. The constant support of the body's total weight in motion is obvious. How it is managed effectively from leg to leg is the refined skill of Yinyang walking.

Optimally it would be best to see your teacher daily to study and practice. Although with students' full work load and family commitments, attending a weekly class to learn and developing a personal routine for daily home practice is more realistic. Even though a portion of the class is reserved for group practice, the main agenda is study; **asking questions, learning new movements and principles**, and **receiving correction**. Don't depend solely on the teacher to feed you knowledge, but learn from the teacher how to feed yourself. You need to be able to discriminate and recognize correct from incorrect, before you can actively make the needed adjustments in practice. Don't try to simply do it right, try to find the flaws that are holding you back from continuous advancement. Don't worry about practicing wrong. Wrong is a relative term. Like a baby falling repeatedly until they learn to stand and then to walk, skill is a process, improved by failure.

The objective is for the student to develop their own home practice routine. There really is **no substitute** for these solo sessions and directing oneself in practice. Experience is the best teacher. Recognizing weaknesses in understanding the knowledge expediently leads to actualizing more clarity exponentially in usage.

People who are employees and work a scheduled week are expected to be at work timely and do a good job. Many people, even though they may find it to be laborious at times, find employment of this nature, a form of supervised discipline that keeps them on track. Left to their own devices (self-employed) they may not fare as well. Being our own keeper is a powerful asset. In essence, a good Tai Chi student does not need to be supervised, but takes on the responsibility themselves to study and practice daily. This is what we are really learning. Be a daily warrior.

When we are less than enthusiastic, how can we use our practice to transform ourselves and self-motivate? Emotional blockages and negative attitudes can by more detrimental than physical limitations. The secret lies in developing empathy to help others to help ourselves, cultivating equanimity to see things clearly in our mind.

Improvement simply means over time our Tai Chi skills are constantly changing for the better. At first our struggles are large as we try to **appropriately** perform the form. With deeper understanding and effort, our practice becomes **approximate.** An advanced student is expected to naturally generate **refined** movements consistently. Keep in mind, as students we are constantly **learning new ways** to articulate our bodies and utilize our minds with more efficiency and effectiveness. The work takes place inside the mind and radiates out in the body. Practice needs to be a part of our daily lives. Then it will become a source of our daily strength.

Before studying the multiplicity of joint articulations and the continuously changing body alignments that must occur to produce refined balanced movement, that we refer to as transitioning, it may be best to look at any movement as a static posture or shape. Initially in our study of a "moving form" practice, we simply use our own understanding of movement and go from posture to posture or shape to shape.

By knowing from a visual standpoint what the correct **finished** posture of Ward-Off Left should look like, we create the proper **starting** posture for Ward-Off Right. The student must gain the ability be able to evaluate the correctness or incorrectness of each posture themselves before any further advancement can be achieved. For example, knowing the external alignment requirements for a front stance; front foot straight, rear foot 45 degrees, heel shoulder's distance, weight distribution 70 / 30, etc., the student can then begin to search for the flaws in transitioning from posture to posture where the errors are manifested and make the necessary corrections. It is important to realize, even though we cannot physically do the form correctly in performance (body usage), we must have the **correct knowledge** and **visualization in our mind**. Finishing the opening posture, how can we begin to learn proper transitioning, if we are not clear what the next posture, Ward-Off Left requires?

Simply expressed, before movement studies can advance, a student needs a clear knowledge of each posture's requirements. Each posture represents the end of a Yinyang cycle and the beginning of the next. Each posture is like a pearl on a string right next to each other. Each pearl must be valued. The thread stringing the pearls together is the skills required to create "continuous movement without interruption". Externally it is easy to just keep the body moving, but it is the application of the internal skills (The 10 Essentials) that forms the intention behind our practice.

A functional posture is not a fixed held position. It is a moment in time of continuous movement. Stances are created by the direction of the waist, shifting the centerline and redistributing the body's weight. An important point is, in a front stance the ability to stand on the front leg (example: preparing to Strum the Lute) or stand on the back leg (Step Back to Repulse the Monkey) should always be accessible even though the form's choreography at the moment does not require it. Stances need to be universal. An unfortunate issue of form practice is incorrectly short cutting one movement because the next movement is anticipated. Don't rush and drop steps. The intention of form practice is to improve body usage. Not to force the body into standard shapes, but to learn how to slowly train the body to change in articulation to "be the form". Continuously paying attention to each movement is essential.

In Yang Chengfu's 10 Essentials # 9, we are advised to "Link (energy /movements) without interruption". Obviously anyone can continuously move their body, so that is only the external requirement. The objective is to connect the various parts of the body (5 bows) together in movement. This is the only way the energy from the root can move effectively and uninterrupted to the hands. Taiji is not aesthetic dance, but a means to issue energy from the body as in pushing and pulling.

Apart from the short pause at the end of each movement in the form (not an interruption or disconnection of Qi flow), there is only continuous movement. **Movement is constant change**. The body is constantly making gross and minute articulations to meet the requirements, so that each movement can store and release energy. Refined movement results in less loss and greater generation of force.

If the body is constantly moving, where is the stillness? Substituting the phrase **consistent stability** may be better words to understand stillness in motion. Obviously in everyday walking we are supporting our body weight on our legs all the time or else we would be constantly falling. Although, how well this is being accomplished is the very point of practice? We often experience the fault of not maintaining the balance (an unintentional change has occurred) when we overextend (weight in toes), lean back (weight past heel edge), or tighten the body, pulling ourselves off our base of support (feet on the floor). **Stillness in Motion is a refined moment by moment consistent stability (central equilibrium - balance) that fosters an appropriately constantly changing frame (the whole body). Motion in Stillness is a refined moment by moment constantly changing frame that does not disrupt the consistent stability (balance).** A symbiotic relationship.

Incorrect articulation destroys balance. Poor balance destroys articulation.

We practice slow with an even tempo to monitor the changes occurring in the body. Responding appropriately at the right time is advantageous. Being early or late in articulation means the timing or coordination is off. Using the waist as the **director of all movement** simplifies the choreography's coordination. The feet and legs energizes the waist. The waist energizes the upper body via the spine.

There are no fixed postures. As beginners, we use our knowledge of movement to simply go from shape to shape. As we advance, through study we realize the form is one long transition. Each movement is a complete cycle of Taiji (Yinyang power). An expression of storing and releasing energy. There is no stopping, retarding, or trapping the energy. Like swimming and staying afloat in water, swim freely in the air with the feet firmly planted on terra firma. You are Taiji.

形 Xing is form. 像 Xiang is image. Form is a tangible physical object. Image is a cerebral "mind construction" (perception) that contains the information we know or don't know concerning a form. The physical practice of Internal work (内家 Nei Gong) is directed by the mind's knowledge acquired through study. The mind creates a picture and this image defines the body's form. For better or worse, image is the mind's reflection of reality. Traditionally in China to develop a student's ability to observe and copy, initial practice is conducting by following along to the teacher's performance. Often no verbal direction is offered. These free public classes are used to glean dedicated participants for future enrollment as students. It is often debated to what significance understanding Chinese culture plays to a student's ability to learn Taiji. While I was attending a Taiji symposium, two masters offered different views. The first speaker emphasized the necessity of understanding Chinese culture (I Ching, Analects, Tao Te Ching, Nei Jing, etc) to comprehend the mind behind the Taiji form. The second speaker stated it was not culture, but modern physics that was more useful in understanding the form in application.

A major consideration in deciding the direction of study and practice is the student's desire to pursue therapeutics or martial application. Clearly the external standard of the form will stay the same, but the internal dimension, which directs expression, will vary. Certainly over time, a student's ambition can change. A natural progression is warrior, healer, sage. A Warrior's study and practice may be modeled after Guan Gong, a famous General known for his Wu De (Confucian martial code of conduct) and the fictional myths found in the literary classic, Romance of the Three Kingdoms. The Art of War by Sun Tzu is commonly thought of as the definitive work on military strategy and tactics. Today it is applied to business. As a civil martial artist, participating in demonstrations, tests, and competitions replaces the life or death engagements on the battlefield faced by the military martial artists of the past.

A Healer would need to pursue a scholarly study of Traditional Chinese Medicine (TCM). Mainly the modality of Qigong therapy and how it applies to Taijiquan energy transformation. The Huangdi Neijing compiled by the mythical Yellow Emperor is the fundamental doctrinal source of TCM. The book, The Web That Has No Weaver by Ted Kaptchuk is a good source to enter this fascinating study. Intimacy with one's own energy is critical to working with the dysfunctional energy of others.

The Sage in China is associated with the three big religions; Confucianism, Buddhism, and Taoism. Seminal classic texts include the Analects, Tao Te Ching, I Ching, and the Dhammapada. Taijiquan becomes a physical liturgy to improve mental and physical health to endure the required long periods of still meditation, chanting liturgy, sparse conditions, and sometimes harsh practices to reach enlightenment. Zhang Sanfeng, Taijiquan's mythological creator was a Taoist immortal. Just as the ancient masters looked toward their past and the latest discoveries in the art and sciences to make their craft applicable in their time, we must do the same. Sir Isaac Newton who is known as the Father of Modern Science was actually the last wizard of alchemy. He believed he was not discover anything new, but unearthing knowledge that was lost to the past. It is believed while searching for the Philosopher's Stone (a material that could change base metal into gold and rumored to be the key to immortality) he went mad from inhaling the toxic gases from his chemical experiments. Likewise, many Chinese alchemists died from the ingestion of quicksilver (mercury) and lead, thought to be key ingredients of the pill of immortality (Dan). Thus the internal school looked toward refining the body's natural transformation of air, water and food into the elixir of longevity (Dan) using Qigong, while the external school experimented with the Earth's bounty of plants and animals to find medicines to cure illness and restore health.

Cheng Man Ching, a student of Yang Chengfu warned that students do not continue to advance simply because they do not stick to Taiji principles in their daily practice consistently. It is important to understand that the various movements found in the hand form are variations of using the body with clear and specific skills. The 5 Skills of shift, pivot, stand, step, and transfer (energy through the body) are the same for each movement of the form. Fusion of the 5 Elements; rooting to the Earth, expanding upward (Fun Kai), deep relaxation downward (Song), expressing energy outward (internal expansion and external extension), and one-point concentration (internal condensing and external contraction) are actualized continuously throughout the performance of the 5 Skills.

Focused awareness, to pay close attention to arising physical sensations relative to each skill in movement, is a means to stick to principle. Experiencing loss of central equilibrium (imbalance), ease (increased stiffness), range (greater restriction), tempo (inconsistent speed), and mental intention (emotional confusion like frustration that affects the body in movement) are clear indications of flaws that need to be addressed before further advancement will result.

In terms of standard choreography, viewing each movement as different will not lead to a consistent body usage. Defining each movement by identifying it as one, several or all of the 5

Skills and fusing the 5 Elements together will reduce movements down into clear Yinyang relationships, and eventually into one complete whole body and mind Taiji expression.

Study is to question practice. Practice is to verify study. As a student advances their understanding of Taiji principles needs to grow continuously just as their physical skills clarify. Study is based on the Tai Chi Classic. This is a loose canon of written teachings passed down through the generations. The Essence of Tai Chi Chuan, The Literary Tradition by Benjamin Pang Jeng Lo is a good source. Armed with an engaged practice and inquisitive nature, illuminating these writing offers a direct connection to the past masters. Teachers employ Skillful Means (Sanskrit: Upaya) and turning phrases to pass information from their mind to their student's mind.

Practice devoid of dialogue, mutual questioning and answering, and academic research and study results in a superficial understanding. The richness of the principles is found in the study of Yinyang (Taiji). Adhering to their practice daily will not only produce superior skills, but open doors to limitless advancement. Taiji practice is easy when a clear path is established. Challenges are met with a mind that seeks resolution. Principles provide answers. Practice makes theory real.

太 极 拳 Taijiquan (Grand Ultimate Boxing) is a martial art that is taught through a form of choreographed fighting techniques. Keeping with the fighting strategy of this school, "overcome hardness with softness" (yielding) and "overcome motion with stillness" (economy of movement), the form is performed slow and relaxed with special attention to deep breathing, balance, ease of joint manipulation, and extended range. The mind's focused intention on body articulation creates a method of moving meditation fostering awareness in present reality.

It is these qualities that attracted an audience not interested in fighting, but seeking therapeutic exercise for both body and mind to improve health, prevent illness, supplement medical treatment, attain longevity, socialize, and feel good.

氣 功 Qi Gong (Intrinsic Energy Work) is a form of exercise often practiced alongside Taijiquan. The main focus is improving respiration through restoration of breathing to full natural functionality. Unlike forced increased aerobic building exercises like running, Qi gong is engaged with the same qualities of performing the Taijiquan form. Although where Taijiquan is a martial art teaching movements that amplify practical skills like pushing and pulling, used in daily life as well as fighting, Qigong is purely exercise, so the movements can explore extended ranges like squatting down low and bending over touching the toes. The extremes of Qigong improve the practicality of Taijiquan.

內 功 Nei Gong and 外 功 Wai Gong are Internal and External categories of Qi Gong. Nei Gong is the soft aspect of Qigong. Wai Gong is the hard aspect. The Taijiquan form is the yin / soft aspect of Taijiquan study. Taking the martial track of Taijiquan study, engaging with another person and expressing energy is practiced in a two-person exercise called Tui Shou (Push Hand). Here the practitioner learns to apply the strategy to the fighting applications of the movements found in the form. Push Hand and Free Sparring expresses Taijiquan's yang / hard aspect. Actual fighting, in its crudest form, relies on excessive muscular force and exhausting aerobic movements to defeat an enemy. As a refined art of fighting, Taijiquan uses mind over matter to attain its strategy. Contrary to this, extreme externalists harden their bodies using a Qi Gong method called Iron Shirt. The body is conditioned to withstand direct blows. Many hard methods produce very effective warriors (like our modern sports warriors; the professional football player), but the detrimental effects of these types of training on health in the long term may be very serious.

As a therapeutic track, practitioners mainly focus on the hand, saber, and sword forms. Although engaging in a safe controlled form of Push Hand offers numerous insights that furthers the student's skills actualized in form practice. It should be noted, Taijiquan totally devoid of its martial root will certainly lack the practicality that is applicable to everyday life tasks. Even though a student may not desire to become a martial artist, having a teacher that is, is a valuable asset.

Beginners often remark they find the movements awkward and difficult to perform. The standardized movements are based on refined natural body articulation, but due to habitual misuse and neglect, many people's bodies do not operate optimally. They become so accustomed to their dysfunctional usage that it becomes their natural. The objective is not to force the body to meet the standard requirements, but to study how the body works correctly and apply this knowledge to practice. When sticking to principles of proper movement, mistakes will occur identifying the flaws. Once recognized, these weaknesses can be addressed. It is important to learn Taiji right because as the common expression points out, it is harder to fix. This is due to the fact that through repetitive practice flaws are solidified.

Appropriate Practice

Start by memorizing the movements as shapes. Use your existing natural body movements for now. Memorize the name of each movement and as a sequence defined as the Five Skills: Shift, Pivot, Stand, Step, Transfer. Many movements will contain all five. Some only a few. This is setting a foundation for practice. There is no substitute for daily home practice where the student self directs their actions. The more time you waste remembering a crude performance of a movement, the longer it will take until the attention can be focused on learning the second practice where proper articulation and adhering to Taiji principles become...

Approximate Practice

At this point, scholarly study becomes a means to advance practice. A study of Yinyang theory applied to Taijiquan and the memorization of Yang Chengfu's 10 Essentials is highly suggested. The mind leads the body. If the mind is not enriched, it has no new perspective to draw from to foster learning. Practice becomes a rote going through the steps. A Yang Zhen Duo Laoshi recommends, taking up a different theme each time practice is engaged will over time cover all the different aspects eventually cumulating in whole body movement with clear mind direction. The student must display in movement that Yinyang is clear before polishing can evolve to a consistent...

Refined Practice

To reach this level, many years of consistent effort have passed. Attending seminars with Yang Jun Laoshi are an imperative. Earlier participation in the ranking system has now brought the student to a level that becoming a teacher is within reach. Daily practice is a way of life. The way is clear. The path is bright.

Although group practice yields benefits, there is no substitution for our daily self-directed solitary home practice. This is personal time to practice and cultivate, focusing on our unique strength and weaknesses.

Apart from socializing with friends, class time is specifically for...

asking question.

From a regular engaged practice, question will spontaneously arise. As past lessons are digested and mixed with new lessons, over time new perspectives and epiphanies will continuously clarify and correlate your knowledge. Taijiquan is a mental study that directs physical practice. To this end, as you advance as a student your ability to comprehend and fully explain the theories and principles related to the practice of Taijiquan is essential. Fundamentally, we are the teacher that teaches ourselves.

assessing current skills and corrections.

To learn more efficiently, we must learn how to self-correct. Even though we may not be able to perform correctly, if we can recognize a mistake or flaw when it materializes, we have the ability to change for the better. During class when the teacher is watching the class's performance and making individual corrections, pay attention. Often another's flaw helps us evaluate our own practice too. Additionally, this momentary correction must be brought into your daily practice or it will simply be repeated later, if corrective measures are not implemented. Often a correction in one movement may be applicable to many others. It is important to take correction in a positive light. Big flaws are external, obvious to the teacher, and usually easy to explain and resolve with determination. As we advance, the flaws may be smaller, more internal, harder to explain, and root out. The work gets more exacting.

learning new material.

When learning new material, simply start by focusing on memorization. Starting with a clear basic shape in the mind sets the groundwork to take the knowledge home. During your home practice, questions should arise. Bring these questions to the next class to seek further clarification. Don't think, "I've got it". This will only limit your depth of understanding. The Taiji form is limited in regard to the number of movements, but it is the quality of each move that we seek to advance by learning more specifics to bring to our daily practice. At some point you will have been taught all the movements. This is when the real work to learn begins.

A priority to study and practice is Cultivation. We cultivate ourselves as a means of personal growth. In our desire to achieve our goals and obtain what we desire, we may force the situation, leading to frustration, anxiety, and stress. The main objective gets suppressed. Cultivation is a means to practice in a way that is consistent to the person we envision ourselves to be futuristically, until such time these qualities are expressed naturally. "Proper practice prevents poor performance."

Although there are many positive personal qualities we may aspire to possessing; being patient, generous, loyal, honest, compassionate, etc. in our Taiji practice we stress two important points that are conducive to cultivating other perfections.

A Tranquil Mind

There is a saying, "The way we do one thing, we do everything." If you are the type that consistently races through your day, pushing just to get things done with little regard to the finer details, truly you are missing the forest for the trees. An opposite effect is having so many things to do in mind, feeling overwhelmed, and accomplishing very little. These are the types of daily minds we seek to address and correct through practice. If our objective is to be less stressed out and relaxed in life, our practice must be in accordance. Taiji is easy to learn, hard to fix.

As a martial art, Taijiquan is classified as a refinement of external (physical) expression. It is called an internal practice because as a warrior, the mind is the major focus of practice. By developing equanimity, facing an adversary with a calm clear mind is advantageous to directing a relaxed responsive body. "Fear of failure" in itself is a major obstacle. Learning to not overreact (panic) when problems arise in our execution and respond appropriately (adjust) is a good example.

Breathing exercises are a means to unify the mind and body. "Regulating the Mind" means by focusing its attention on the correct object of perception, the proper state can be maintained. Often referred to as the Qigong State or associated with the psychology of Flow, with practice, a deep concentration fills the mind's reality.

When extraneous thoughts enter into the field of awareness, a trained mind will not indulge these momentary tangents, and refocus. As a moving meditation practice, a one-point concentration practice can be brought to every aspect of our life. Dealing with the present moment fully, even during adversity, can be greatly enhanced by utilizing a mind of equanimity developed by proper practice. Tranquility in practice is interrelated to the next point, A Relaxed Body.

A Relaxed Body

Optimal body usage does not mean limp, like the extreme of slouching on a couch or the other extreme, standing stiff like a soldier at attention. The first example is called collapsing; the joints are too closed, not providing proper upward support. The other example, opening / expanding the body is overextended. The joints are fixed and locked open. The body is pulled upward losing its Earthly root.

We say, "Curved, but not curved" to express the concept that the joint is closed too much, making extension difficult. We say, Straight, but not straight to express the concept the joint is locked open making flexion difficult. These extremes cause the body to lose relaxation. The joints are forced into tight dysfunctional ranges.

When muscles are relaxed deeply, the expression, "Let the meat hang on the bone" is applicable. The bones act like a frame connected together by ligaments. The muscles via the tendons do not pull the body's structure out of alignment. The lower body feels heavy and expressed as "Sink the body" as the body weight drops through the legs and feet into the floor. Tightened muscles trap the weight in the body. Due to the fact muscles are energized to tighten them, "Sink the Qi (energy) to the Dan Tian" (lower abdominal area) is an expression to say, by relaxing, the energy is turned off that is trapping too much tension in the muscles. Often when articulating the body in a choreographed manner, the new and challenging movements bring with them a lot unnecessary tension.

The mind and the body are one. When we are committed mentally, without considering the logistics of the body, this forced mental intention will cause physical tensions to rise simultaneously. How we use the body also affects the mind. Especially when the movement is fast and with momentum. Practicing slow and accurately is to learn how to relax deeply, so faster movements can be performed with greater efficiency. Study at a slow pace allows the mind ample time to see and comprehend the full range of movement, instead of directing with quick broad polarized intentions.

It is important not to lose the spirit of cultivation in practice. Tranquility of mind and relaxation of body should not be mistaken for a laissez faire attitude. The object is to not be burdened with extraneous thought, to see essential reality, and absorb deeper into the present moment's engagement. The body under a mind's clear, calm direction will not be adversely physically affected. Consciously, taking what is gleaned in daily practice into every daily activity will strengthen attainment.

Tai Chi is taught as a system. Although the hand form comprises the major aspect of practice, to actualize the theories of Yinyang as principles in the body and mind, other supplementary exercises are employed to clarify the three areas of study; Body, Breath, and Mind. These areas, indivisible as the entire body in function, isolated in study and practice, will lead to a synthesis of a greater refined whole.

Body: Here initially we mainly focus our attention on learning the choreography. When reproducible on an appropriate level, a long term study of human movement is applied to an equally long term practice. Taking the time to research on a deeper level, simply by beginning to view anatomical medical pictures of the skeleton, will clarify how bones are connected. Furthering investigating muscles, ligaments, and tendons will provide a clear picture in the mind to how they are utilized in articulation. For instance, in Yang Cheng Fu's Ten Essentials (which is the center of our study) number 2 states, "Contain the chest, Raise the back". This is a simplistic statement that requires a clearer "internal vision" to actualize as refined movement.

Breath: Often an associated exercise to Tai Chi, Qigong (Energy Work) is included in practice. This is primarily a system that focuses on improving respiration. The whole body is essentially comprised of energy (matter) in different states, that survive off the oxygen absorbed from inhaling air and exhaling waste (carbon dioxide). Considering oxygen is more important to sustaining life than nutrition and drinking water, daily breathing exercises should be given greater priority. A large amount of the toxin formed in the body is gathered and expelled through the breathing cycle.

Meditation: This is to directly see the mind in operation. The practice can be performed lying down, sitting, standing, and walking. The practices can be both static and dynamic. These practices reduce mental stress by improving concentration. Learning to focus naturally on one point continuously, and weakening the pull of extraneous thoughts, that continuously arise in the mind leading the attention astray, results in achieving a deep relaxation of both body and mind. Staying in the present (reality), the objective is not to try to stop thought, but direct its intention.

The main point is, each of these three areas of study, focuses on one topic of practice. Meditation focuses on the Mind. The meditation posture is fortified by dynamic and static body practices (Tai Chi form, Post Standing, and Qigong). The breathing, which is a typical meditation focal point, is improved by the respiratory practices found in Qigong. Thus, meditation practice itself is not the appropriate time to focus on improving body usage or breath quality. The meditating mind utilizes the breath and awareness of the present moment (being in the body here and now) to unify the body.

During body practice, (Post Standing and Tai Chi Form) focus the mind on the movements. Choreography, Five skills, joint alignment, relaxation, upward expansion, monitoring the rising and falling of various physical sensations that may signal imbalance or excessive force are examples of the numerous themes that can be selected to address the body in movement. Refining the quality and quantity of breathing should be addressed during Qigong, just like the mind advances during the engagement of meditation practice. Again, the point is to practice with a clear intention. More like a horse with blinders plowing a straight row without variant than a monkey jumping here, there, and everywhere.

Finally, Qigong is respiratory in nature. Postures are fortified with Body practice. The mind with Meditation practice. This approach, of clear Body, Breath, and Mind practices lead to a clarification of "Three in One". Regardless of what we do physically or mentally, the whole body unifies from the greater refinement in these areas.

For students who are committed to making this a lifetime study and practice, here is an approach that will yield decades of themes to explore in even greater depth. Each area of practice is now expanded upon.

Post Standing / Tai Chi Form = Body-body / Body-breath / Body-mind

Qigong = Breath-body / Breath-breath / Breath-mind

Meditation = Mind-body / Mind-breath / Mind-mind

Prior each area of study focused on that specific area. Now each area is practiced focusing on the other areas, forming 9 studies.

Armed with the refinement gleaned from the individual areas of study, the Tai Chi Form can function better as a practice to improve the body, breath, and mind. These are the internal trainings that can then be externalized for those who choose the martial track. For those on a therapeutic track, the functional nature of body usage in Tai Chi will externalize in common daily tasks like squatting, lifting, pushing, pulling, walking, sitting, etc. As meditation, the martial artist will glean a mind of equanimity, that will maintain a relaxed attitude in a dangerous environment. As therapy, stress is reduced as a physical, energetic (breath), and cerebral clarity emerges with the establishment of a Center. The Center (aka Middle, Waist, Lower Dan Tian) is the focal point of all three areas of study that ultimately unifies the body together with greater clarity.

Week 48 - Baby Steps

All fields of academic study or trade crafts have a vast wealth of knowledge, collected over long periods of time, that is passed down, revised, and expanded upon by successive generations. As students we seek teachers that are in possession of this information and seek their direction on how to obtain it for ourselves. We must acknowledge that this knowledge can only be passed along incrementally in small digestible pieces. All too often, students "know" more about a subject, than they can demonstrate in application. This can cause confusion and stagnation.

At seminar, Yang Jun Laoshi spoke on this point. This is my understanding of his remarks. In the east, students tend not to question the learning objectives of their teacher. They trust that they are be presented with information in a timely manner that leads to efficient understanding and practice. Teachers are not holding back information. The student is required to demonstrate that they absorbed the lesson, prior to receiving more guidance. Often the teacher asks, and the whole class responses back. Reciting, following, watching, and listening are vital skills.

Westerns, tend to need a lot more verbal explanation, before they will engage. More collateral knowledge is requested, pertaining to the lesson, but far exceeding the priority of the moment. Tangents like, why do we do it this way, and not that way? Here the student has not even learned one way yet, and wants to debate another method. It makes the lesson broad and the objective to be met less direct. It is my opinion, a common hurdle to be overcome is to not overfill our mouths (smaller bites) chewing on too much food at one time, and not swallowing enough to digest the lesson. Literally, forcing too much information down our throats.

Regardless of beginner, intermediate, or advanced status, learning should be seamless and ceaseless. The same topic can be addressed at different levels. The words "Basic Training" in many people's mind refers to instruction for beginners. Possibly substituting the idea "Essential Training" would be closer to the definition of Basics used in Tai Chi. An advanced student is a practitioner who consistently and naturally demonstrates refined Basics. To achieve this, it is imperative to cultivate a study and practice that is founded on a patient, tranquil, relaxed, daily, and determined approach with short and long term goals.

I encourage my students to read, research, and watch videos, but be careful not to get the "cart before the horse". Therapeutically, this is a self-paced track with attention focused on addressing specific health oriented concerns. If a student aspires to becoming a teacher and enrolls in the certification process, then they must fully commit to a timelier scheduled motivated pace of practice.

Due to its slow methodical pace and emphasis on relaxed articulation, Tai Chi is very safe compared to active exercises like running and aerobics. In practice, we never force the body to conform to the Form's Standard, which is based on correct natural body usage, but we understand that the untrained body needs to transform over time to attain ease and greater range of motion. Being clear in the mind first, to how the body needs to articulate to perform a specific choreography, is what makes Tai Chi a "mind directed practice". The mind's attentiveness to the body's sensations creates a feedback loop. The mind commands the body with an Intention and then the body relays back vital information to what is actually occurring. Problems occur when the Mind's Intention forces its will upon a body that gets no attention.

As a healer to ourselves, we must observe **Primum non nocere, First do no harm.** In the early 1970s when Tai Chi was just getting discovered by the American masses, doctors were reporting injuries from its practice. This was possibly due to misinterpreting the instruction or simply going through the form and lacking the proper attention. Although, Tai Chi in its initial stages is very reflective to how a person routinely uses their body. Considering one of the therapeutic features of Tai Chi is improving balance and strengthening the core and legs, through the practice of standing and pivoting on one leg to a much greater extent than the limited motions most people perform during an average day, done improperly with too much force and hast can be the real source of the problem.

To avoid knee complications, pay close attention to these points:

Knee Over Toe

Often it is how the teaching is classically presented than is the issue. It is best to think that the knee should not go past the toe. If is aligned properly over the ball of the foot / metatarsal. In a properly formed front stance, looking down a student should be able to see a portion of the toes. The shin is not ninety degrees in relationship to the floor, but angled. Overall, what is important to understand, the weight of the body must pass through relaxed, not locked joints to be able to provide the correct upward support (as in Newton's third law of motion). We shift into stances. They are not fixed postures. In aligning the knee in motion this is usually where the second concern arises. We use the performance of the form as a venue to understanding how the body needs to function to perform a desired movement. We need to change the way we use our body to improve, not just go through the motions more times. A single correction may take persistent work to resolve.

Shifting, not Lunging

In shifting forward in a bow stance, the rear leg is the power, and the front leg is the major support of the torso; eventually bearing seventy percent of the body's weight. Instead of creating the upward support by properly articulating the front leg, the knee movement is erroneously more forward lunging in the direction of the rear legs expression of power. This also takes place when shifting backward. Here the knee instead of seeking alignment over the knee is dropped down toward the floor collapsing the stance. Like a house' frame that drops the roof's weight into the foundation, a properly formed stance will carry the torso in movement with much less muscular tension and energy waste.

Rotate the whole leg when pivoting to fix the foot position.

Making an analogy of the leg as an archery bow, because it only flexes and extends naturally in one direction, it is the "articulation of joint" mainly in the pelvis / femur connection that aligns rotates the knee and ankle in the desired direction of usage. Improperly done, the knee experiences a torque; a twisting inward or outward with excessive tension. Notably this is similar to the rotator cuff in relation to the arm.

Full and Empty

Full is when all the body weight is on one leg. The other leg being completely empty of body weight is called Empty. Think of the Empty leg like an empty vase. It still retains its shape. A common problem, when shifting to stand on one leg takes place, when the empty leg collapses and loses it shape. The knee is no longer aligned in its intended direction prior to stepping, but may be pointing off course. A lot of problems with knee alignment may be solves, if the order of leg articulation in stepping is clear; Waist moves the hip, hip moves the thigh, knee moves the shin, ankle moves the foot. Like the arms also, articulation is sequenced from the center out. Doing Tai Chi by leading with the hands and feet is not adhering to the principles.

In conclusion, it is this author's opinion that knee injuries are not caused by Tai Chi, but may accelerate a negative condition because proper body usage is not explored and utilized. Instead the student continues to use their body, in a manner that they perceive to be correct because it feels natural, when in fact it feels natural because they simple got use to using their body in an inferior way. Tai Chi is not difficult to learn, if care is taken to see with new eyes and be attentive to what the body is trying to communicate to the mind. Hear yourself. Listen closely.

In archery, a target is brought into sight and the arrow is aimed. This is an analogy to first establish a clear desired objective (Intention) in the mind and then find the means to hit the target using the body.

Tai Chi Form practice is classified as a Yin Internal exercise. A major characteristic of this method of exercise is maintaining a soft (relaxed) body and mind. This conforms to the Tai Chi Principle: "Softness overcomes Hardness" This is to use as little force (undue muscular contraction) as possible to animate the body, by removing any restrictions to its ease and range of motion during articulation. This can only be achieved when the mind is softened. A hard mind is not open or responsive. Its tunnel vision and obsession to hit the target tightens the body.

Although it is a common perspective to separate body and mind, the flesh from the spirit, the brain is a physical organ of perception. The mind's calm (relaxed) awareness can monitor the body's reactions more efficiently, to its direction of the body's movement and offer appropriate and timely corrections. Both the body and mind must be relaxed. The mind must listen to the body's reaction to its direction by feeling and responding to physical sensation. Conversely, the body must be trained to respond accurately to the mind's intentions. **There is a big difference between not being aware of the body's actions, due to not paying full attention, and not being able to perform an action because the skill has not yet developed to a sufficient level.**

Tai Chi is a "mind directed" exercise. Developing a strong, clear, realistic Intention in the mind through study, that is applied to the body during practice, is to aim and shoot at the target. **To refine, we must be able to identify flaw and work patiently to reach its resolution.**

The second characteristic of Internal exercise is a slow even pace of body movement. This relaxes muscles and offers the mind ample time to experience the ever changing bodily sensations leading to better mind direction. This conforms to the Tai Chi Principle: Stillness overcomes Motion. This is a study of economy of motion and the realization that often a small adjustment (correction) in the body has a profound affect in dynamic expression. Like shooting the moon, a little off on Earth is a lot off course in space.

Combining "Slow and Soft" the practice emphasis is on refining intrinsic energy (Qi) that is produced by relaxation, deeper breathing, balance, ease and range of motion, joint articulation and alignment, coordination, and tranquility of mind.

External exercises are done more robustly because increase speed and muscular engagement brings the energy out in expression. Usually these exercises are defined as resistance training, which helps to keep the muscles healthy and strong. Making the tools part of the body is sought through proper practice. Saber, sword, and spear training fall into this category too.

Week 52 – Emotions

Encountering ourselves when learning new things or trying to do things differently, especially under the direction of another, can bring up a lot of unsettling emotions. Generating unnecessary expectations may cause our anxiety to grow, making a peaceful situation stressful. Forcing a change, instead of cultivating patience and allowing natural growth, may be an old bad habit reapplied again from the past. Often the way we do one thing, we do everything. Slowing ourselves down and relaxing is the method for creating an interior environment conducive to learning both in the mind and the body. Our mantra, Tranquil mind. Relaxed body.

How we practice mentally is just as important, or even more so, to how we practice physically. Mind leads the body. Our attitude (Shen - Spirit) may need an adjustment first. Ten minutes of static seated or standing meditation using abdominal breathing can be just the medicine (Dan) to move the energy of the mind down, out of being trapped in a labyrinth of thought in our head, into the vast silence of the body, deep in our Center (Waist). We are learning how to transform destructive energy (from internal or external sources) into creative energy. We need to make positive affirmation expressed in speech, our thoughts and actions. Actions can speak louder than words, but words become as monuments to thought.

It is very important to disassociate, doing something correct or incorrect, from the disruptive emotional states that may arise from being good or bad at what we do. If our actions don't live up to our expected outcome, we need to focus on "why" it went wrong by continuing to cultivate a peaceful mind. Frustration or even worse, anger will only destroy the very relaxed body we are trying to cultivate in our practice. Conversely being overly satisfied with a minor achievement, may cause us to think "we got it" and proceed to nest comfortably, resting on our laurels, stagnating the possibility of further advancement.

In the performance of the Tai Chi form it is suggest the face should remain serene in appearance. Concealing the emotions is to "conceal our hand" as in card playing with a poker face. It would be best if the outside matched the inside. That is the purpose of training. Although, acting accordingly is the path to actualizing accordingly. As in group class, it is considered very bad form to bring our personal frustrations out into the class. Our actions should not disturb the tranquility of mind and relaxation of body of our fellow classmates. Again, acting accordingly is the path to actualizing accordingly. This is not to say, suppression is the answer, but bringing our problems up privately would be more appropriate. Students should also consider, Tai Chi is not a substitute for psychological or physiology treatment from licensed therapists and doctors. Dealing with problems correctly is part of practice.